Healing Therapies
for
LONG COVID

"Long Covid—after an initial Covid infection or post-vaccination exposure to spike proteins—is an unpleasant experience that affects almost every organ and system in our body, brings us down with a wide range of symptoms, and activates several dormant infections. Using his broad education, research skills, and innate intuition, Vir McCoy expertly combines tips and techniques from alternative and mainstream medicine and creates a protocol with a distinct 12-step goal that could turn us into effective healers and free us from the grip of long Covid. In the chess game of Covid versus humankind, this book shows us how to become strong winners."

VATSALA SPERLING, PH.D., AUTHOR OF *THE AYURVEDIC RESET DIET*

"Vir McCoy approaches health and healing with no preconceptions as to what modality is best. Vir encourages you to tap into your own intuition to be your own best healer. Follow your own inner guidance with this book, tap into the resonance of your body, and see where it leads you. It is the best skill we can have for the times we are in."

ANGELICA LEMKE, N.D., AUTHOR OF
HEALING COMPLEX CHILDREN WITH HOMEOPATHY

"Vir McCoy has been a perfect example of how we as healers, no matter the credentials we have, can learn from our patients and bring their gifts forward, integrating their discoveries and applying their vision to others. Vir makes it ever more legitimate to work as a team, doctor and patient, with compassion on both sides, and the wisdom of intuition—so important in the art and practice of healing. Thank you, Vir, for this outstanding work at this most necessary time."

DANIEL BEILIN, O.M.D., L.AC.

Healing Therapies
for
LONG COVID

An Integrative and Intuitive Guide
to Recovering from
Post-Acute Covid

VIR McCOY

Healing Arts Press
Rochester, Vermont

Healing Arts Press
One Park Street
Rochester, Vermont 05767
www.HealingArtsPress.com

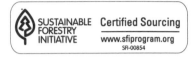

Text stock is SFI certified

Healing Arts Press is a division of Inner Traditions International

Note to the reader: *This book is intended as an informational guide. The remedies, approaches, and techniques described herein are meant to supplement, and not to be a substitute for, professional medical care or treatment. They should not be used to treat a serious ailment without prior consultation with a qualified health care professional.*

Cataloging-in-Publication Data for this title is available from the Library of Congress

ISBN 978-1-64411-778-1 (print)
ISBN 978-1-64411-779-8 (ebook)

Printed and bound in the United States by Lake Book Manufacturing, LLC
The text stock is SFI certified. The Sustainable Forestry Initiative® program promotes sustainable forest management.

10 9 8 7 6 5 4 3 2 1

Text design and layout by Virginia Scott Bowman
This book was typeset in Garamond Premier Pro and Gill Sans with Trenda used as the display typeface

To send correspondence to the author of this book, mail a first-class letter to the author c/o Inner Traditions • Bear & Company, One Park Street, Rochester, VT 05767, and we will forward the communication, or contact the author directly at **VirMcCoyHealth.com.**

. . . .

Disclaimer on How to Use This Book

Although readers may find these exercises, medicines, practices, and suggestions useful, they are made available with the understanding that this book arose out of the author's personal experiences and are not meant to diagnose, treat, cure, or prevent Covid-19 or any other illness. The author is not a doctor and presents only his own experience. Individuals afflicted with Covid-19 should engage in a program or treatment with a licensed qualified physician or other competent professional. Readers should consult a physician in matters relating to their health, particularly concerning any symptoms that may require diagnosis or medical attention.

. . . .

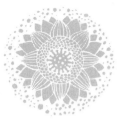

Contents

Appendices

My Intuitive Healing Journey with Long-Haul Covid

THIS BOOK AROSE OUT OF MY JOURNEY with long-haul Covid, or post-acute sequelae of Covid (PASC). Before I became sick with Covid, I was healthy and active. I surfed, ran, swam, did yoga and breathwork, and exercised regularly. I considered myself health conscious and in touch with what worked for my body. I ate a mostly organic diet with high fats, few grains, lots of vegetables, and tons of herbs and wheat-grass. I had plenty of love in my life, no real stress, lots of meditation, and so on. But that did not protect me from what was to come.

My first symptoms of Covid-19 came in early December 2020. It was likely the Alpha variant, and pre-vaccine. I likely contracted it at Thanksgiving that year, as I had a few folks over, although no one else got sick.

My initial symptoms were mostly mild, with some body aches and a low-grade fever for three days. After about a week I noticed I had lost my sense of smell, which tipped me that my illness might be Covid. I tested positive by PCR test on December 8. Except for the loss of smell, the initial symptoms soon abated.

However, a couple weeks later other symptoms kicked in, with headaches (which felt like an ice cream headache or hangover that wouldn't resolve), brain fatigue (which felt sort of like an electrical-frizz brain fire), loss of smell, lethargy, weakness, general malaise, ringing in the ears, mild cough, sleeplessness, anxiety, air hunger, jumbled thinking, and depression. Later I developed a kind of mental "fritzing," or scrambled brain, like I was going crazy, plus blurry vision in my right eye. In addition, I suddenly developed a histamine intolerance, or mast cell activation syndrome (MCAS). High-histamine foods that had been healthy mainstays in my diet for years, like sardines and fermented sauerkraut, had to be eliminated. Sometimes consuming just one high-histamine food would trigger an excruciating headache that lasted for days. It turns out many others were experiencing symptoms that were very similar. This was what was being called long-haul Covid.

There were times when I was in so much pain for so long that I felt like giving up, as I know some do. The mental scrambling and the pain were almost unbearable at times. Chronic pain can grind a person down and create depression, but I knew I had to keep the faith and ride it out for the "long haul." I had too many people I loved, including my newborn child, so I just had to keep going and get well.

In Los Angeles, I found a doctor who practiced integrative medicine and was experienced with long-haul Covid, and I also consulted with two doctors, Stephen Harris and Runa Basu, who'd been incredibly helpful when I was recovering from Lyme disease in years past. Blood and urine tests showed an increase in cytokines and inflammatory markers, increased glucose levels (to the point of being prediabetic), increased levels of the C4A protein (common in cases of chronic infection and inflammation), exposure to high levels of mold (aflatoxin and others), low testosterone levels, low levels of CD8 and CD57 lymphocytes, high cholesterol, increased levels of Epstein-Barr virus antibodies, and other weird things like low uric acid and cortisol levels. These all turned out to be classic long-haul indicators.

In addition to the M.D.s, I also went to herbalists, acupuncturists, homeopaths, osteopaths, Chinese medicine practitioners, neuroplasticity retraining (the Gupta Program), and various hands-on and energy healers. As those with long-haul Covid know, you will do *anything* to get better. Sometimes it was incredibly frustrating, with waaaaay too many pills and expenses. But I kept at it and eventually narrowed it down to what was working for my body.

After a month my sense of smell came back. Slowly but surely, over the course of a year, I got better. I took notes on my progress and insights. I read all the research I could lay hands on, looking for evidence to support my own evolving understanding of the disease and its treatment. As I progressed, I slowly began to put together a protocol for treating long-haul Covid, with the guidance and feedback of doctors and healers.

That protocol became the basis for this book. There was no miracle cure; instead, what worked to help me recover from long-haul Covid was a comprehensive integrative program that included both Western and alternative medicine, a dietary regimen, psychospiritual development, mental and physical activities, and *time*—it's not a quick process. Though I worked with a variety of medical and therapeutic experts, much of my healing journey was directed by what may seem an unlikely guide: my intuition.

I have always been sensitive to sound and energy, even as a child, in a way that seemed a bit unusual. These sensitivities and a love for nature directed me into the fields of natural science, art, and music. I now work as a field biologist and botanist, conducting rare plant and animal surveys, as well as a professional musician, touring venues and music festivals throughout North America. I have worked at both of these crafts for more than thirty years.

A third career developed along the way. I had struggled with health issues as a teenager and in my early twenties, which led me down the healing arts path. I went to massage school and later obtained certifications in somatic and neuromuscular therapies. Over the years I also studied herbology, breathwork, meditation, homeopathy, and various other healing modalities.

From 2001 to 2009, I was sick with Lyme disease. During that time, I began to "see" inside myself the way a shaman or medical intuitive might.* I began to have sensory impressions or insights into what

---

*When I speak about intuitive insights, I often use the word *see* (or something similar) in quotation marks. This implies that I am using the word in an intuitive sense and not in the literal sense.

was going on inside my body, and remedies and things my body needed to heal came to me, like the way a dog craves grass or other animals seek out other specific plants when they are sick. These sensory impressions, or suggestions as I call them, provided a window into the appropriate path of healing for my body, an ability I believe we all possess. I call it intuitive access, and I believe it is an important tool for healing for all of us. I coauthored a book with Kara Zahl about my experience with Lyme disease called *Liberating Yourself from Lyme* (Healing Arts Press, 2021). Learning from and learning how to use intuitive access constituted a major part of my healing and thus constitutes a significant part of both of my books. Where relevant and appropriate, I have drawn from the earlier book.

The intuitive process involves quieting the mind and tapping in to our sensory perception. We all get a "hit"—that gut feeling about something—from time to time. It may come in the form of an image, a smell, a sound or word, or a feeling that seems to arrive from beyond us. That's our intuition working, and it is a powerful tool for healing and navigating in the world. Accessing that inherent intuitive power comes from a relaxed, loving place. A place of *listening*. There are exercises in this book to help you cultivate this tool and build your intuitive muscle.

Most of the remedies presented in this book came from explorations I undertook using this intuitive process during my illness. I kept listening to the pain, tuning in to my body, trying to figure out: *What is my body telling me? What is the matter? What does it need?* The process was both humbling and validating, teaching me to trust my intuition. When I was "shown" a remedy, I would read through the latest medical research or check in with my doctors about it, and they would confirm and refine what I had intuited. This method helped me validate what I was seeing and sensing.

Though I rely on my intuition for direction, I have no intention of debating against science. In fact, it's the opposite: I believe the scientific process is essential for collecting information and validating (or not) what we intuitively hypothesize. The intuitive process is a kind of spiritual science, like an inner Sherlock Holmes looking for clues. You get a lead (from intuition), and you track it down to confirm it (with science).

The protocol I developed for the treatment of long-haul Covid, based on a partnership of intuition and science, is broadly integrative, combining the common and the unusual. It includes not only my own intuitive information but also many promising options, protocols, and remedies from other success stories, with the science to back them when available. Some suggestions and medicines are of an anecdotal and unproven nature, but it is important to know what has worked for others, and sometimes science takes a moment to catch up to validating (or disproving) what may appear to be effective.

I rarely write about dosages in this book, as it is extremely important to work with a professional for that. If a medicine or remedy is potentially toxic or may have a bad reaction with another medicine, I note that as so. A hodgepodge of pills may work against you, and one person's remedy may be another's poison, so always proceed with utmost caution, and again, work with a qualified practitioner to determine the dosages and regimens that are right for you.

With long-haul Covid you must find the middle road: Work with a good integrative or functional doctor or healer who understands long Covid, and trust the intuitive process. It's important to find a doctor or healer who has all the tools in the kit, from Western to alternative, because you're likely going to need them all.

As well, don't be afraid to reach out to others for support and connection. Long-haul Covid can be incredibly debilitating. We are not meant to take it on alone.

Cracking the long-haul Covid code has been an incredible group effort among scientists, doctors, practitioners, healers, and people like me, searching for answers. Much more information continues to be uncovered. It is my hope that this book teaches you not only to trust your intuition and unique path but also to find the remedies, practices, and practitioners that work for you. Ultimately this book is meant as an offering to help you find a way through the suffering a lot more quickly than I did, because long-haul Covid is not fun—not fun at all.

✦✦

This book is not a substitute for a doctor, but hopefully it is a useful tool to help you see not only what I intuited, as a guide, but also what you may intuit. Becoming your own medical intuitive is incredibly powerful. After all, it is your body, and ultimately your willingness to listen and heal, that will guide you. Hang in there; there is a way through.

∽∞∾

ACKNOWLEDGMENTS

Thanks to my wife, Heather Christie, and to my father, David McCoy. Thank you to the works of Dr. Bruce Patterson, Dr. Mobeen Syed and the Front Line COVID-19 Critical Care Alliance (FLCCC), Dr. Angelica Lemke (who was consulted for the Homeopathic Repertory for Covid Symptoms included in this book), Dr. Michael Hirt, Dr. Runa Basu, Dr. Dan Beilin, Rick Williams, Stephen Harrod Buhner, the amazing staff at Inner Traditions who helped bring this book to life, the Gupta Program, angels, guides, masters St. Germain and Quan Yin, nature spirits, all the folks belonging to Survivor Corps and many other long-haul support groups, fellow long-haulers like Susi Love, and the amazing scientists and healers working together to help heal long-haul Covid.

1

✦ ✦ ✦

Long-Haul Science

Predispositions, Etiologies, Symptoms

OUR SCIENTIFIC UNDERSTANDING of long-haul Covid is still emerging, with many doctors, scientists, and patients racing to find answers. By the time you read this, new information on how the disease develops will have become more clear, and breakthroughs in treatment may have occurred. However, the etiology of long Covid is now fairly well researched and understood, and this book includes more than 350 scientific references along with options for healing that have helped many, but most importantly, helps teach *you* to find remedies for your own body.

What follows is a general overview of the nature of Covid-19, and it is designed simply to offer a basic understanding of the disease. For more comprehensive information, look to the references cited at the end of the book and the growing body of research available online.

ACUTE COVID: VIRAL INFECTION

Coronavirus disease 2019 (Covid-19) is caused by the SARS-CoV-2 virus. This virus consists of replicating RNA enclosed in a lipid membrane. The outside of the membrane is coated with spike glycoproteins (chains of amino acids with a sugar coating). The spike proteins—specifically the subunit of the proteins labeled S1—allow the virus to access cells in the host body by locking into the cell receptors for angiotensin converting enzyme 2 (ACE-2), which are found mostly in the gut, heart, and brain (Medina-Enríquez et al. 2020; V'kovski et al. 2021). The resulting viral infection triggers inflammation.

> *My initial infection with Covid was mild, but I remember a distinct feeling that the virus hit me in the gut first. Early on, I had a clear vison of my gut being torn up, like tiles from a floor that had been pulled up. I "saw" the virus in my meditations, and I "heard" the sound of a machine casting a metallic object over and over: "Kachunk, kachunk, kachunk, kachunk . . ." It sounded like a replicating little metal bug. Is the virus alive? Most scientists say no; some say maybe; I would say just barely.*

It turns out that Covid-19 disrupts the gut microbiome, which plays a crucial role in the immune system (Burchill et al. 2021). A preexisting gut imbalance can contribute to the severity of the infection (Yeoh et al. 2021). It's like Covid disables the army in your gut first, then goes and wreaks havoc in the rest of the body. Sneaky little beasts. So, the gut then becomes a key place for healing. (We will discuss rebuilding the gut in chapter 4 and chapter 6.)

Acute Covid cases that are mild or asymptomatic occur in approximately 80 percent of cases, and severe cases (requiring hospitalization or causing death) occur in approximately 20 percent of those infected with Covid (Verity et al. 2020). Severe cases are often associated with underlying conditions, age, and ethnicity factors, often involve the lungs, and often require hospitalization (Luliano et al. 2022). However, these statistics have shifted with the increase in new variants like Delta, Omicron, and the BA strains where the death rate is less than with the Alpha and Delta strains.

Severe acute Covid can cause neurological disorders, microclots, brain bleeding, stroke, vascular and neurologic inflammation, encephalitis, encephalopathy, epilepsy, pulmonary issues, neurodegenerative diseases, organ damage, and much more (Achar and Ghosh 2020). A cytokine storm takes over, overwhelming the body, and can cause permanent organ damage, including in the brain (Hojyo et al. 2020).*

> *Acute Covid left me with permanent kidney damage (about 25 percent loss of function), and I suspect that long-haul Covid caused some brain damage as well. Fortunately, the brain has plasticity and can heal around damaged areas, as we shall see.*

PROLONGED VIRAL PRESENCE

According to some studies, actual competent viral replication with the Alpha variant twenty days after the onset of symptoms was possible, but unlikely. There are, however, documented cases of prolonged viral RNA shedding, with detectable levels lasting two and a half months (Turner et al. 2021). Moreover, a recent paper (preprint at the time of this writing) found replication-competent virus up to 230 days after the onset of symptoms (Chertow et al. 2021). However, most researchers currently tend to suspect that long-haul Covid is a disease not of a replicating virus but of the fallout or "trash" from it.

LONG-HAUL COVID, OR
POST-ACUTE SEQUELAE OF COVID (PASC)

Many researchers consider long-haul Covid, or PASC, a different disease from acute Covid. Acute Covid is an infection by a replicating virus, whereas PASC is a disease of chronic inflammation arising from the damage to blood vessels and organs by leftover viral debris (spike proteins) of the virus (or spike proteins from the vaccine; see page 8), coupled with a malfunctioning immune system and autoantibodies gone haywire.

---

*Cytokines, which are cell-signaling proteins, will be further discussed later in this chapter (see "High Cytokine Levels" on page 12).

Long-haul Covid is loosely defined as having symptoms lasting three months or more after infection. Long-haul symptoms can differ from those of the initial infection; the condition can arise even in a patient who was asymptomatic during infection. They can include:*

Difficulty breathing or shortness of breath
Tiredness or fatigue
Symptoms that get worse after physical or mental activity
   (post-exertional malaise)
Difficulty thinking or concentrating (brain fog)
Cough
Chest or stomach pain
Headache
Tachycardia
Joint or muscle pain
Pins-and-needles feeling
Diarrhea
Sleep problems
Fever
Dizziness upon standing (lightheadedness)
Rash
Mood changes
Change in smell or taste
Changes in menstrual period cycles
Hormonal disruption
Thyroid issues
Increased glucose levels
Mental disruption and psychiatric issues
Hair loss
Blurry vision

---

*This list derives from Mehandru and Merad 2022. Dr. Roger Sehuelt offers an excellent summary of long-haul symptoms in a lecture for the MedCram Coronavirus Series (update 129) on YouTube, posted on June 21, 2021, under the title "Long COVID Treatment, Symptoms, and Recovery (Long Haulers)."

Cataracts

Increase in other "bugs" (e.g., Epstein Barr, herpes family viruses, mold infections)

And much more!

Conservative estimates made in August 2021 placed the number of cases of long-haul Covid at more than fifteen million (Phillips and Williams 2021). Studies in 2022 showed that 20 to 40 percent (or more) of Covid cases, whether mild or severe, may develop into long-haul Covid (Groff et al. 2021). These numbers were likely specific to the original Alpha strain; however, there are many reports (at the time of this writing) of the Delta and Omicron variants causing long-haul Covid. Long-haul Covid occurs not just adults but also in children, and in not just in the unvaccinated but in the vaccinated as well (Buonsenso et al. 2021; Massey, Berrent, and Krumholz 2021). A long-haul or persistent Covid syndrome can last for months and even years (Lopez-Leon et al. 2021). This whole scenario results in immune dysregulation and gene changes (Marx 2021). In a survey conducted in June through August 2022 aproximately 15 percent of people who had Covid were still dealing with long Covid, some for more than two years (Centers for Disease Control and Prevention 2022).

In my case, when asking my body intuitively why I had long-haul Covid, I clearly "heard" the word genetics, and I got a "hit" that my previous experience of having Lyme disease had set up a hypersensitivity in my immune system. (This was before I had read anything about this.) Previous to infection with Covid, my blood tests showed normal levels of Epstein-Barr virus antibodies, glucose, testosterone, cholesterol, immune cells, and vitamins and minerals. I had had no real Lyme disease symptoms for more than thirteen years and had tested negative for that disease many times over that duration. In short, I was just fine prior to Covid. We will see shortly how Covid can disrupt the homeostasis of the body and stir up latent "bugs" like Lyme.

Let's turn now to the evidence for predispositions to long-haul Covid, the two main working theories of the etiology of this disease, and other symptoms and issues that arise from the corresponding inflammation. Note, however, that this discussion is by no means comprehensive, and new studies will shed more light.

Predispositions

Many potential predispositions to PASC are just being discovered, but they can include diabetes, obesity, diet, gut dysbiosis, imbalanced vitamin and mineral levels, high stress and hypertension, elevated triglyceride and cholesterol levels, impaired insulin production and higher levels of glucose, inflammation, previous infections, presence of Epstein-Barr and other viruses, autoimmunity, exposure to toxins like molds, imbalanced blood proteins and other biomarkers (like decreased CD8 T cells), and much more (Palmos et al. 2022; Papadopoulou et al. 2021; Masana et al. 2021; Huang et al. 2021). We discuss some of these factors later in the book.

Researchers have also discovered a number of genetic or DNA factors that may indicate a predisposition to acute Covid and PASC (Pairo-Castineira et al. 2021). In addition to others, it appears that Neanderthal DNA may play a role. One study found that having higher levels of Neanderthal DNA resulted in a greater chance of severe Covid (Zeberg and Pääbo 2020); conversely, some Neanderthal DNA seems to protect us from Covid as well (Zeberg and Pääbo 2020). The genetic risk aspect may offer some explanation for studies showing that many seemingly healthy people, including children, can develop PASC (Thomson 2021).

> *Interestingly, I myself have higher levels of Neanderthal DNA, as determined via a 23andMe DNA test. (I think I learned this when I ate some magic mushrooms one time, but that's another story.)*

Etiology
Lingering Spike Proteins/Viral Debris
Studies have found a common culprit in Covid long-haulers: lingering viral spike proteins. One study led by Dr. Bruce Patterson found that

in long-haulers, the nonreplicating Covid S1 spike proteins cross the blood-brain barrier and persist inside a type of white blood cell called nonclassical monocytes. These nonclassical monocytes normally patrol blood vessel walls and can be found all over the body. In a published study conducted by Dr. Patterson and his team, among a group of people who had developed Covid early in 2020, persisting spike proteins were found lingering inside nonclassical monocytes up to fifteen months after the initial infection (Patterson et al. 2022a).*

Another study conducted with Covid-infected mice found a similar result: lingering spike proteins causing immune dysregulation (Colunga Biancatelli et al. 2021). And in another small study of sixty-three Covid long-haulers, spike proteins were discovered in the blood in a majority of subjects up to twelve months post infection (Swank et al. 2022)

Spike proteins can do great harm in the body. For example, studies have found that the spike protein can damage the heart and mitochondria as well as gene expression (Avolio et al. 2021; Yang et al. 2022).

In long-haul Covid, the nonclassical monocytes carrying the lingering spike proteins attach to blood vessel walls via CCR5 and fractalkine receptors, causing microtears, plasma leaks, and microclots, which lead to elevated cytokine levels and vascular inflammation (Pretorius et al. 2021). Interestingly, CCR5 is the same receptor that HIV uses, and there is similarity between some proteins in HIV and the Covid spike protein (Wu Zhang and Leng Yap 2004). Dr. Patterson and his team used CCR5 and fractalkine antagonist drugs (receptor blockers) to stop the monocytes from attaching to receptors, thereby stopping or slowing the inflammation (see chapter 7 for more detail).

---

*This etiology of long-haul Covid reminded me of Lyme disease, where you deal with similar "persistor cells" that cause all sorts of dysregulation and irritation. However, I believe Lyme keeps *replicating* in the form of dormant cysts that can hatch and cause a flare-up. In this way, Lyme is more like a chronic infection, while long-haul Covid is more like a backed-up sewage system clogged with nonreplicating viral debris (spike proteins).

> *In my intuitive meditations I have "seen" the spike proteins inside my body. To me they looked like colorful Tinkertoy pieces, but one thing stood out: they were as hard as rocks. They even looked like little rocks or grains of sand. They were like trash that would not break down; backing up and creating a clogged sewer. I had a moment where I was "scanning" through the spike protein itself and found the tiniest bit of intelligence, as if it had just a wee bit of programming in it. And that turns out to be somewhat the case; researchers have found that the Covid virus can mutate its spike proteins so that antibodies don't recognize them, thus evading the immune system response (Weisblum et al. 2020).*

With lingering spike proteins, antibodies respond to the antigen-presenting nonclassical monocytes (white blood cells), adding to the fray with an immune system in hypersensitive overdrive. It's like the nonclassical monocytes with the spike proteins stuck inside them are saying to other immune cells, "Help! There is something in me, come get it!" But there's a problem: the spike proteins are inside the same white blood cells that tried to clean them up in the first place. When other cells come to the rescue, they may end up attacking those monocytes, setting up an autoantibody or autoimmune situation, as researchers have discovered. This sets up a massive inflammatory response. It is like some of us are simply allergic to the spike proteins.

Post-Vaccine Long-Haul

With the mRNA vaccines, a "script," or messenger RNA, is created in a lab and directs cells to form spike proteins in the body to help create antibodies. In this way the vaccine teaches the body to recognize and defend against Covid. Normally the body makes the antibodies to Covid and cleans out the remaining spike proteins.

However, in rare cases, the vaccine can trigger symptoms similar to those of long-haul Covid. In an analysis of more than 17,000 long-haulers, Dr. Bruce Patterson and his team found that about 1,500, or 10 percent, of long-haulers never had Covid but did have the vaccine (Patterson 2022a). These post-vaccine long-haulers had something in common with post-Covid long-haulers: spike proteins inside nonclassical monocytes, months after administration of the vaccine. In a study (preprint at the time of this writing) fifty post-vaccine long-haulers had their blood studied (Patterson et al. 2022b). Using high-tech PCR, viral genome sequencing, and "machine learning," Patterson and his team were able to observe single spike proteins inside the white blood cells (nonclassical monocytes).

The researchers theorize that the immune system sends monocytes to break down the vaccine-initiated spike proteins, but just as happens with Covid, the proteins get "stuck," like a splinter or grain of sand, inside the cells, and they persist, potentially triggering the development of long-haul symptoms.

There are other new (as of this writing) studies and preprint reports emerging indicating a post-vaccine long-Covid symptomology that is basically the same as long Covid, including autoimmune disease and vaccine-induced neuropathy (Waheed 2021; Safavi et al. 2022), circulating spike proteins in the blood after vaccination (Ogata et al. 2022), immune cells spreading spike proteins from the vaccine (Seneff et al. 2022), and vaccine-associated myocarditis (Mansanguan 2022).

Post-vaccine long-haul is likely less prevalent than Covid long-haul; studies indicate that the total exposure to spike proteins from the vaccine is less than that arising from actual infection (Heinz and Stiasny 2021). In many cases (including my own) the vaccine can actually help alleviate long Covid symptoms. In a large study of long-haulers this was found to be the case. Vaccinated subjects experienced increased recovery compared to unvaccinated long-haulers. Symptoms were lessened or in some cases completely resolved (at least temporarily), perhaps by triggering the immune system to recognize the spike proteins (Ayoubkhani et al. 2022).

• •

Autoantibodies/Anti-idiotype
Antibodies/Autoimmunity

Autoimmunity is a common characteristic of long Covid; in fact, it has become a hallmark indicator of Covid (Rojas et al. 2022). The exact mechanism or trigger, however, is still being researched. According to Dr. Patterson and others, the persistent spike protein is the culprit.

In an attempt to narrow down the potential mechanisms of Covid infection, vaccination reactions, and long Covid, an assessment of clinical observations published in the *New England Journal of Medicine* proposed the network hypothesis as a possible explanation. This hypothesis describes an autoimmune-like response in which the body produces antibodies to a specific antigen and then also produces antibodies to those antigen-specific antibodies. These secondary autoantibodies or anti-idiotype antibodies, as they're known, attack the body's own immune defenses.

In the case of Covid, the authors suggest that the body makes antibodies to the spike protein, but in some cases the body may also then make new antibodies that attack those antibodies (Murphy and Longo 2022). These autoantibodies also attack the ACE-2 enzyme that helps regulate the immune system as well as white blood cells (likely the nonclassical monocytes with spike proteins) and other cells (Arthur et al. 2021). The autoantibodies also cause blood clotting and microtear damage (Shi et al. 2022). This scenario is similar to that of autoimmune diseases like lupus; in fact, it's possible that this auto-antibody response to Covid may mimic or trigger other autoimmune diseases (Zamani, Moeini Taba, and Shayestehpour 2021). Similar autoimmune responses have been observed in the cerebral spinal fluid of Covid patients, which may help explain some of the longer-lasting neurological symptoms (Song et al. 2021).

In my intuitive meditations I "heard" the word malfunction in reference to my immune system and "saw" crossed wires in my brain. This suggested to me that my body was having a hard time dealing with the Covid viral "trash." I also very clearly "saw" bloody clots and tears in the blood vessels, with scabs attempting to heal over them.

The damage from the initial infection, lingering spike proteins in the nonclassical monocytes, and autoantibodies can trigger a cytokine storm and inflammatory reaction with myriad symptoms, such as ringing in the ears, hair loss, rashes, heart palpitations (tachycardia), neurologic issues, lymphatic stagnancy, psychiatric conditions, and much more (Conti et al. 2020; Nalbandian et al. 2021). So neutralizing these autoantibodies becomes important, as does breaking down or removing the spike proteins.

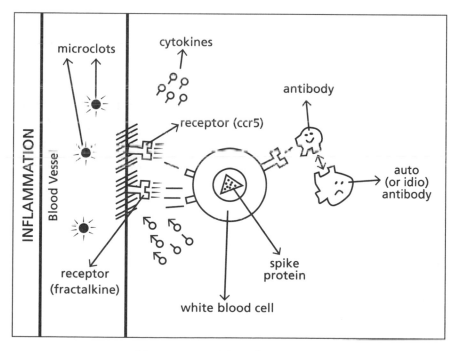

Monocytes with spike proteins

Symptoms

High Cytokine Levels

Cytokines are proteins involved in cell signaling. The immune dysregulation caused by lingering Covid spike proteins and autoantibodies, as discussed above, can cause a large increase in cytokines. These small proteins are secreted by cells of the immune system, including macrophages, B and T lymphocytes, and mast cells, and they modulate immune responses and regulate the maturation, growth, and responsiveness of particular cell populations. They include chemokines (CC), interferons (IFN), interleukins (IL), lymphokines, and tumor necrosis factor (TNF), among others. Types of cytokines that may reach abnormal levels in long-haul Covid are TNF-alpha, IL-2, IL-4, IL-6, IL-8, IL-10, and IL-13. Other cytokines and receptors involved with long Covid may include GM-CSF (granulocyte-macrophage colony-stimulating factor), sCD40L (soluble CD40 ligand), CCL5 (a.k.a. RANTES), CCL3 (a.k.a. macrophage inflammatory protein 1 alpha or MIP-1 alpha), IFN-gamma, VEGF (vascular endothelial growth factor), and CCL4 (del Valle-Mendoza et al. 2022). Some labs now test for these abnormal cytokine levels and have created a long-hauler index (Patterson et al. 2022a).

The key cytokines that consistently show up with high levels in long-haul Covid are TNF-alpha, CCL5, and IL-6. These cytokines in high quantities cause blood vessels to dilate and literally become leaky. This can create a host of vascular congestion issues, including brain swelling, confusion, low albumin levels, activation of fibroblasts and problems with the skin, increased heart rate, and many other inflammatory issues associated with long Covid.

Many medicines can help reduce levels of cytokines, such as low-dose naltrexone (Parkitny and Younger 2017). We'll explore these medications in chapter 7.

Chronic Histamine Overload:
Mast Cell Activation Syndrome (MCAS)

Mast cells are white blood cells found in the connective tissue throughout the body and mediate allergic reactions. When, for example, mast cells detect an allergen, they release histamine into the bloodstream. Histamine causes blood vessels to expand in order to allow the free flow of other chemicals sent by the immune system to combat the allergen. The increased blood flow causes inflammatory symptoms such as heat, redness, and itchiness.

Mast cell activation syndrome (MCAS) is an immunological condition in which mast cells inappropriately and excessively release these chemical mediators, resulting in a range of chronic symptoms. These symptoms are prevalent in long Covid, and they can include fatigue, brain fog, shortness of breath, ringing in the ears, joint pain, headaches, and more (Weinstock et al. 2021). According to some mast cell specialists the root of MCAS is actually mold in the body.

> One indicator of MCAS is that eating foods containing histamine worsens symptoms. That was true for me; I developed allergy-type reactions to histamine-containing foods within a few weeks of having Covid. I had never experienced that before. If I ate the wrong food, like sardines, whammo! Massive headaches sometimes for days. (We'll explore diet and medicines for calming this reaction in the following chapters.) I also had a "download" that I had become allergic to my own blood.

Vascular and Neural Inflammation

The initial Covid infection can cause organ and tissue damage and corresponding inflammation in the nervous system and vascular system. With long-haul Covid this creates a chronic state of post-infection inflammation and a corresponding variety of symptoms, such as hair loss, skin rashes, swelling, back pain, and more.

> In my intuitive meditations, I "saw" images of bombed-out buildings, with blood cell damage, microclots, and smoking embers, as if a fire had raged through my brain.

Vagus Nerve Impairment and PTSD

The vagus nerve, which is the longest nerve of the autonomic nervous system, becomes impaired because of the chronic inflammation with long Covid, resulting in dysfunctional brain-stem signaling (Dani et al. 2021). In addition, the sympathetic nervous system, which mediates the fight-or-flight response, gets stuck in a kind of post-traumatic stress disorder (PTSD) loop of alarm stemming from the limbic system and amygdala (Tu et al. 2021). (We explore methods for healing these symptoms in chapter 5.)

Cortisol and Hormone Disruption

Covid causes inflammation of the pituitary gland in the brain, which leads to hormonal disruption, including reduced levels of cortisol, which regulates, among other things, the stress response and blood sugar levels (Umesh et al. 2022; Klein et al. 2021). These and other hormone imbalances can cause low testosterone levels in men and irregular menstrual cycles in women. Blood tests often show these hormonal imbalances in long-haulers (Frara et al. 2021; Wang et al. 2020).

Activation of Other Infections

With Covid, previous immune dysregulation from infections like Lyme disease and herpes family viruses like Epstein-Barr and varicella (shingles and chicken pox) may be stirred up and can complicate the situation, or even become the new problem (Liu, Sawalha, and Lu 2021). Candida infections and mold sensitivities can also flare up. It's like the immune system is so taxed with Covid that any bug under the surface gets a "get out of jail free" card, and then they go wreak havoc. This flare-up of EBV and other herpes family viruses is common with long-haulers (Gold et al. 2021).

POTS

Postural orthostatic tachycardia syndrome (POTS) is a blood circulation disorder characterized by rapid heart rate increase when standing.

The vascular inflammation associated with long-haul Covid can trigger this syndrome (Raj et al. 2021).

Mitochondrial Imbalances

Mitochondria are organelles that serve as a cell's primary source of energy production in the form of adenosine triphosphate (ATP). In the event of an infection, mitochondria contribute to immunity by engaging the interferon system and inducing programmed cell death (apoptosis). In cases of severe or chronic Covid infection, the mitochondrial energy production system suffers, and the mitochondria can be hijacked and severely damaged by the virus, creating more inflammation and cytokines. Defective mitochondria can also cause an iron buildup, increased coagulation, and greater cell death (Ganji and Reddy 2021).

> *Certain supplements like NAD and antioxidant-rich foods become important for scavenging the "trash" of the virus. I had many visions of blueberries, blackberries, pomegranates, garlic, oils, and more.*

Neurological and Psychiatric Effects

Research has shown that even mild cases of Covid can cause permanent structural changes in the brain (Douaud et al. 2022). Long Covid has been shown to cause mental illness, shrinking of the brain, confusion, and a kind of psychosis and derangement of thoughts and dreams (Naidu et al. 2021).

> *When I was at my worst, I remember feeling anxiety and panic because my brain no longer worked properly. A very real mental instability crept in, with scrambled thoughts. I can see why some people with long Covid check themselves into psychiatric care facilities. The psychiatric symptoms can be debilitating. I found that fluvoxamine, a selective serotonin reuptake inhibitor (SSRI), helped me considerably with this, and it has been found to be of great benefit for other long-haulers as well (Lenze et al. 2020).*

Fortunately, the brain has a measure of plasticity, meaning that it can repair itself or create new neural connections to circumvent damaged areas (Mateos-Aparicio and Rodríguez-Moreno 2019). Drugs and herbs that support cognitive ability and brain health come into play here, especially the medicinal mushrooms, like lion's mane, reishi, chaga, and turkey tail, and microdosing with psychedelic mushrooms (Sabaratnam et al. 2013; de Vos et al. 2021). (We will explore these remedies in chapter 5.)

Gut Imbalances

Imbalances in the gut may influence the severity of inflammatory symptoms (Liu et al. 2022). But they can drive chronic illness as well (Lazar et al. 2018). And Covid itself can disrupt the gut, including the balance of specific flora, such as bifidobacteria, levels of which have been found to be low in long-haulers (Bozkurt and Quigley 2020). (We'll look at a number of issues that can underlie this imbalance, including diet, emotions, and energetic balance, later in this book.)

Tinnitus and Vision Impairment

Long Covid can affect the vestibular and cochlear nerves, causing chronic vertigo and ringing in the ears (Malayala and Raza 2020). In addition, neurological and hormonal damage can manifest as blurry vision and develop into cataracts, a symptom seen in many long-haulers, including myself (Hu et al. 2022).

> *I had consistent ringing in the ears throughout my experience with long-haul Covid. I "heard" the word* vestibular *and "saw" the plant iris. Turns out, Iris versicolor is a good homeopathic remedy for ringing and buzzing in the ears.*

Gas Imbalance/"Air Hunger"

"Air hunger" is a common long-haul symptom. Indeed, Covid patients may have lower levels of carbon dioxide (hypocapnia) and oxygen (hypoxia) in their blood (Hu et al. 2021; Geier and Geier 2020). (There are breathwork exercises that can help this; see chapter 3.)

> *I often had images of gas bubbles, the smoke from a bubbly water (carbon dioxide), and oxygen tanks in my intuitive meditations.*

Glymphatic System Overwhelm

With all the "trash" of the Covid virus and dying cells in the body, the lymphatic and glymphatic (cerebral spinal fluid) systems get overwhelmed and backed up, causing soreness in lymph areas in the neck (Bostancıklıoğlu 2020).

> *The back of my head, along the sides of the occiput, was always sore and I had images of dirty bathrooms, clogged sewage systems, and piles of trash. This was the most consistent image I had: rotting spike proteins and trash, and I always had images of soaps and detergents to break this down (more about that in chapter 9).*

· ·

Exercise

Exercise can exacerbate the symptoms of long Covid by increasing white blood cell counts and ramping up the immune system (Geraghty, Hann, and Kurtev 2019). Normally that boost in immune function is considered one of the benefits of exercise, but in the case of long Covid, that's exactly what we don't want. We want a *calming* of the immune system.

· ·

ANALOGIES

An Army

The acute Covid infection, whether mild or severe, storms through a body. It's like an army invading your town, with soldiers inflicting all sorts of damage on the infrastructure of blood vessels, neurons, and cells and laying spike mines in the streets. Everywhere you see smoldering fires, damaged buildings, and debris. The immune army then marches in to break down and clean up everything. However, in some people the immune soldiers find that they can't disarm the spike mines (they were not trained for this), some soldiers get confused and don't recognize the spike mines, and some soldiers end up looking like the spikes. The immune system ramps up and calls in its special forces teams to come help. The new soldiers are confused by the situation. They kill the old soldiers and start zapping innocent civilians as well. The immune system in a sense becomes allergic to its own blood, attacking the spike "zombies" that it thinks are going to come back to life. Chaos reigns. Now, while the guard is down, other "bugs" that were in prison, like Epstein-Barr virus and molds, escape and wreak havoc as well. As debris and dead soldiers accumulate, the medics and cleanup crew become overwhelmed. The town's streets fill up, creating more inflammation and stagnant blood and lymph.

A Car
It's like the immune engine is racing but not in gear. You shift into drive and hit the gas hard to get moving, but someone poured sand (spike proteins) into the transmission and the gears are stuck. The car bucks and jumps as the engine floods with gas and backfires, clogging up the exhaust with pollution.

A Chronic Allergy
The offending allergen is the spike protein, and your body is caught in a chronic allergy, remaining in a state of histamine and inflammation.

SUMMARY
Drivers
In addition to predisposition, whether genetic or not, there appear to be a number of factors pointing to the drivers of long-haul Covid. The major components appear to be:

1. Damage from the initial infection
2. Lingering spike proteins
3. Autoantibodies/malfunctioning immune system

4. Latent infections from other viruses, bacteria, and molds that flare up
5. Vascular and neural inflammation, which leads to myriad symptoms including hormonal disruption
6. Limbic PTSD—with the limbic system stuck in a trauma loop, the immune system stays in overdrive
7. Backed-up lymphatic and glymphatic system

Goals

The following become our goals for treatment and are outlined in the rest of the book:

1. Decrease inflammation, mast cell activation, and the cytokine storm. In other words, put out the fire.
2. Block or reduce the overactive monocytes and rogue immune cells. Prevent these monocytes from docking/binding at their receptor sites (CCR5 and fractalkine) on blood vessels.
4. Dissolve the spike proteins (and blood clots) with medicines, or reeducate the immune system and white blood cells to recognize and dissolve them or let them go.
5. Calm the limbic system and the PTSD loop/stimulate the vagus nerve.
6. Improve lymphatic and glymphatic drainage and detoxification.
7. Get the gut microbiome in top shape and heal the gut lining.
8. Eradicate any lingering Covid RNA and other pathogenic viruses, bacteria, and molds that have flared up.
9. Heal any underlying emotional and/or ancestral traumas or predispositions (if possible) that may be adding to the dysregulation of the immune system.
10. Help the brain heal with neuroplasticity retraining programs and grow new neurons as in neurogenesis
11. Get the mitochondria working properly again and increase cellular health.
12. Practice patience. Give the immune system time and rest.

2

✦ ✦ ✦

Intuitive Access

An Invaluable Healing Tool

IN THIS CHAPTER, WE'LL SHIFT GEARS from science to what I call spiritual science. If our goal is healing, one of the most important tools we have is our own intuition. Intuition was instrumental in my own healing, and teaching you to use your own, whether to heal from long Covid or any other ailment, is one of the primary goals of this book.*

The following words, which first came to me when I was battling Lyme disease, have been a tremendous source of inspiration over the years and are relevant here.

The Healing Decree of Immunity

Walk in Love.

Walk in Peace.

Ask the Matter,

What's the Matter?

End the Mental Chatter.

Look Closely: What Do You See?

Work with the Physicality

---

*Much of the material in this chapter was drawn from the introduction to *Liberating Yourself from Lyme,* "Learning to Listen."

Bless Your Body
And the Enemy.
Liberate Those That Seek to Harm Thee.
Harm Not Thy Own Body.
Stand Firm against Those That Seek to Harm Thee.
Forgive Yourself from the Past.
Support Your Immune System to Do Its Task.

LEARNING TO LISTEN

In *Liberating Yourself from Lyme,* I told the following story of a powerful validation of my own healing intuition. The time frame and the disease are different, but the intuitive process is the same.

About a year after I was diagnosed with Lyme disease, a spinal fluid analysis showed an increased number of white blood cells in my spinal fluid, and the doctor I was seeing immediately put me on intravenous antibiotics. I went into the hospital every day for forty days, and I would lie in the hospital bed while an intravenous (IV) bag was hooked up to me to receive ceftriaxone, an antibiotic. Lyme had gotten into my brain and was back with a vengeance.

Six months earlier I had finished a course of doxycycline after being diagnosed with Lyme. At the time I thought it was all over, that I was cured. Little did I know it was just the beginning. Lyme had entered my brain, and like a kind of meningitis (infection of the brain) was ravaging my head and body. My brain felt like it was on fire and swollen, and I was moaning, covered in sweat. As I lay in the hospital bed, I began to cry. I was in a state of utter despair. What in the hell was going on? Why was I sick again after taking antibiotics? I began to pray for help, for anyone or anything to show me what was going on, to show me the way.

I could still breathe so I focused on my breathing. Because I couldn't think properly (Lyme jumbles your brain), I began to feel more. *If I can still feel, and I can still breathe, and I can still love, I still exist,* I thought. Then I "felt" into my brain and asked, *What's the matter?* as if my brain were a little baby. Very gently and lovingly, I asked again,

What's the matter? I love you. I felt like a mother who senses something is wrong with her baby, even though the baby can't speak. With all of the love and tender feelings I could muster, I "cradled" my brain and asked again: *What's the matter? I love you, brain. What's the matter?*

Then a miracle happened. I had a vision. I saw a beautiful large oak tree in the woods, and up the side of the trunk, shelf of the trunk, shelf (or polyphore) mushrooms were growing. Rows and rows of these beautiful mushrooms spiraled up the tree toward the sky.

I remembered three kinds. Two I recognized from my work as a field biologist: one type was reishi mushrooms, another was turkey tail mushrooms, and the third I had to wait till I got out of the hospital to look up, but they were called chaga.

I need these, I thought.

The vision was so clear and in a place of love that I knew there must be something to it. Once I was out of the hospital, I researched the mushrooms. It turns out that reishi mushrooms have been used for thousands of years as an immune booster in Chinese medicine. Turkey tail mushrooms are also immune boosters and are part of an anticancer drug currently being developed and tested called PSK, and chaga is another incredible immune booster (Stamets 1999).

A short time later I read in *National Geographic* about Ötzi the Iceman. Ötzi, a 5,300-year-old man who had been mummified in ice, was found in the Alps in 1991 by hikers on an unusually warm day. He was brought to scientists, who examined him to discover how he died, what he ate, and what diseases he suffered from. It turns out Ötzi had Lyme disease (Hall 2011). Reading this nearly bowled me over. Lyme disease, I realized, has been around for a long time, or at least some version of it has. Ötzi wore a belt with a leather pouch, and guess what was in that pouch? Shelf mushrooms like I had seen in my vision: tinder fungus, or polypore (*Fomes fomentarius*), and birch polypore (*Fomitopsis betulina*). Both mushrooms are antibiotic and antiparasitic (Stamets and Zwickey 2014). Then I got chills. I speculated he was treating his Lyme disease with these mushrooms. Whether he had visited a shaman or had intuited this cure himself, I have no doubt he was using them to treat himself. I used the information from the article as validation, confirming my intuition that reishi and shelf mushrooms could help me heal.

I completely healed from Lyme disease by listening to that deeper wisdom and creating a protocol based on my intuition. Medicinal mushrooms, which have become quite popular and are also very helpful for long-haul Covid, became a big part of my healing. Back then in 2004 there wasn't much information about them in the mainstream. It was this powerful intuitive vision that led me down another path. I realized that perhaps the answers are already there, we just have to *access* them. Intuition became a powerful tool in my medicine kit, helping me to heal from both Lyme disease and long Covid.

INTUITIVE SCIENCE

After I got out of the hospital all those years ago, I began to hone my intuitive skills, much like one would practice an instrument or develop a muscle. I began to practice the art of intuitive sensory perception inside my own body and write down what I was seeing, tasting, smelling, and hearing during my meditations. What we call clairvoyance, clairaudience, and so on is, as Carl Jung suggested, the spirit speaking symbolically (Jung 1968).

I would then do research on what I was experiencing and look for the science to validate my intuition. Later I would home in on proper dosages with doctors and practitioners.

THE HOLOGRAPHIC MEDICINE CHEST

Our physical bodies have evolved and adapted on Earth for millions of years. All the plants, animals, and minerals that make up Earth have evolved and adapted along with us. Our bodies are made up of the basic mineral building blocks of Earth and, I believe, are infused with the breath or spirit that animates all life (or however you see it). It is this interface of spirit and matter that many call the soul. Many cultures access this as a place of feeling and being rather than thinking. When you are in this state of your soul, plant and animal spirits and angels can communicate in the form of symbols, images, dreams, synchronous events, feelings, and sensory impressions, which are much more palpable. We need to quiet the mind, relax, and enter into a feeling of love to sense this. Though our ancestors wove it into their daily lives, most of us have forgotten this ancient wisdom and, along with it, the innate ability to know what or how we need to heal. I believe we all have the ability to access this information, though some people are more naturally attuned to it than others. In reality, there is what I call a holographic medicine chest that we all can access. All the minerals, plants, animals, and medicines in and on Earth that have been here for millennia are potential medicines waiting to be discovered.

Though we are more removed from our instincts than animals, humans are still animals with the capacity to know what we need to heal. We can access our intuition through meditation, dreams, movement, breath, relaxation, dance, stillness, and many other healing modalities. A healer can also hold the space and be a catalyst for this exploration as well. Yet all beings possess the ability to be medical intuitives. You must simply look within and be open to all possibilities. Some believe that the best belief system is no belief system at all. Be open to the idea that you have innate wisdom within yourself.

As I believe we each possess this remarkable gift, we need to create the space for the magic to unfold. When you listen to the body's wisdom, the deep messages or sensory impressions of the soul, it can help guide you toward finding life balance. Your intuition can magically show you what can be helpful in your healing. You must be open to listening to these messages from your body, mind, and soul.

THE INTUITIVE PROCESS

We have all had experiences with this, the "aha" moments, the sixth sense, the hits, the downloads, trusting the gut, the guidance, and the intuitive insights into the nature of reality. We can access intuition in the liminal space—that place between the worlds, between the mental and the spiritual. That space we inhabit when we first wake up from sleep. Intuition may come in the form of an image in your mind's eye, a smell, a thought, a word, a sound, a feeling, or a synchronicity. Your sensory perception becomes a window into the body. The body/spirit will show you what it needs to heal, but we have to listen, to quiet the mind.

⚘ *Intuitive Meditation*

Put on some calming music or nature sounds. Lie down and make yourself comfortable. Close your eyes. Begin to take some deep breaths. Breathe in, counting to four. Then breathe out, counting to six. Squeeze your whole body, then let go. Relax.

Feel your feet. Relax them. Soften. Breathe.

Feel your head. Relax your jaw as you exhale. Breathe. Relax your eyes; breathe. Relax your ears; breathe. Relax the back of your neck; breathe. Let go of your mind and relax into your physical body.

Imagine that your head is melting downward, like melted butter, sinking and flowing into your chest and then into your heart, bringing your awareness to this center of love. Observe your thoughts, but give them no energy. Your thoughts are not who you really are.

Now see a flame like a candle in your heart. Feel this heart flame; feel it as your connection to divine love. Think of a thing you love: a pet, a partner, a child, trees, the ocean, snowcapped mountains . . . Keep thinking of what you love until you generate the feeling of love in your heart. Feel how love feels. Feel the burning in your heart.

Take a deep breath. Look now, and look closely. What do you see in your body? Feel into any pain or discomfort with your loving awareness. Bring it into your heart and cradle it. It could be an arm, your brain, your liver, your whole immune system . . . whatever is calling for attention the most. Hold that pain like a mother would hold her baby. Rock it gently. Tell it you love it. Lovingly ask, *What's the matter? What do you need?* Then breathe and listen in the silence. Feel. Follow the stream of consciousness that is your intuition waiting to reveal itself to you. Your body may communicate with you through sensory impressions. What do you see? An image may float into the mind's eye. A plant? A food? An action? An insect? What sensation arises? What feeling bubble up? Be open to anything. Breathe, relax, and listen.

Stay in this place for as long as you like. If your mind wanders, return to the feeling of love by thinking about what you love.

When you are ready, thank yourself and open your eyes.

If anything came to you, write it down in a journal, even if you have no idea what it means. You are looking for clues. Be open to *anything*. Sometimes you may not sense anything except for the pain. That's okay. Practice this meditation again and again. Building intuition is like building muscle—it takes time.

I have found that the best time to do this meditation is in the morning, when you just wake up and are in that subliminal or in-between state of waking and dreaming.

Intuitive meditation is a powerful tool for healing. That does not mean you should abandon your doctors or healers—but with intuition, you have direct access to the deeper wisdom of your own body, right there inside of you, to inform and guide your efforts. You just have to listen.

3

✦ ✦ ✦

Melt the Disease in Love

Finding Your Energetic Anchor

IN THIS CHAPTER WE ARE GOING to go deeper into the energetic component of the disease and the anchor we can use to heal from it: love.*

WHAT LOVE FEELS LIKE

Are you your thoughts? Most of us would say no, that this "I" is something beyond a thinking or mental place. Call it spirit, God, presence, light, love, nonduality—it does not matter. What matters is the feeling. The *feeling* of love. This feeling comes from a place beyond our thoughts. It is our anchor, our home, beyond any worries or stresses. Beyond any illness. It is a field of connection far greater than we can comprehend or describe. It is a place of the infinite, a place of spirit. This place, this connection, is who we truly are. And we become our own greatest healer by anchoring in this feeling of love.

Setting that anchor is not always easy, especially if we are suffering and in chronic pain. Sometimes death can be grace, but we have the ability to access a deep healing when we practice the art of embodied

---

*Love is a powerful medicine for all ills. Some of the material in this chapter was drawn from *Liberating Yourself from Lyme,* chapter 2, "Bless the Enemy."

love. Attachment to suffering and a fear of death only exacerbate the problem. Love is the way out, but it takes practice, surrender, and focus.

What does love feel like? Let's find out.

⚕ Anchor in Love Meditation

Lie down or sit and make yourself comfortable. Close your eyes. Begin to take some deep breaths. Roll your head gently in circles. Take some deep, slow, wavelike breaths, bringing the air deep into your belly and then rising up to your chest. Full inhalation, full exhalation. Relax and let go with each exhalation.

Continue to breathe slowly and deeply. Now soften your jaw. Soften your eyes. Soften the optic nerve that runs all the way from your eyes back into your brain. Soften your ears and the little ear bones. Breathe.

Soften the back of your head (the occiput). Soften the juncture where your spine meets your brain. Breathe, relax, let go.

Bring your awareness to your body. Notice any pain. Just observe it, as if you were only your breath, separate from pain. Breathe. See if you can soften deep in the center of your brain. Imagine that your head is melting downward, like melted butter, sinking and flowing into your heart, bringing your awareness to this center of love. Feel your center of perception—the observer and all thoughts—right there in the center of your chest. Breathe. Begin to think of the things you love. What do you know you love? Mountains, rivers, pets, music, a partner, Jesus, flowers, rain, Mother Mary, Buddha, your grandmother, a friend, trees, the ocean, music, dancing . . . Breathe. Ask yourself: *What does love feel like?*

Imagine a candle in your heart. A flame that never dies. An infinite fire. Let's make it bigger. Think of those you love and imagine sending them love. Pour it out with all your might. Imagine cradling them like babies. Call on your angels and guides to help you amplify that love. Pour it out to them. Breathe. Become the flame inside. Anchor in this feeling.

Say to yourself, "I am." Associate this "I am" with that *feeling* of love. See the candle flame growing larger and larger. See it filling every nook and cranny of your body, melting any disease, anything that is not love. Take a big breath and bow to this love. Let your head surrender to your heart. Adore yourself.

When you are ready, take a big breath. Slowly open your eyes.

Your body may be sick, but your spirit is not. You are not a disease. Your body may be going through a nightmare, but this is not who you are. Return to your breath, and center in your heart again and again as often as you can. Rest in the peaceful, loving feeling you will find there. Be the eye of the storm, the true you, as often as you can. Find the anchor. The way out is in.

⚜ Stop, Drop, Walk

When you are having anxious or depressing thoughts, practicing this exercise can help you find your way out of the cycles of worrying.

1. **Stop.** When you feel your mind spinning out, catastrophizing outcomes or obsessing over symptoms and remedies, you can simply say, "Stop," silently or out loud.

2. **Heart Drop.** Take a big breath and think about the things you love, just as you did in the preceding meditation, and drop your awareness into your heart. Anchor your awareness there in that feeling of love.

3. **Gut Drop.** Now take your awareness and drop it lower into the gut, imagine there is a hot fire or ember there. Stoke that fire by imagining a time when you were in full health and doing something active—skiing, playing baseball, making love, or just going for a run. Bring that feeling of health into the present. Now notice the feeling of heat or fire in your belly. Get fierce; tap in to the warrior within. No stupid little bug is going to take you. Feel how powerful you are. Add some quick breaths of fire to activate the gut even more (see exercise on page 44).

4. **Walk.** Then take three deep breaths and do something else. Distract yourself. Go for a walk, do some yoga, watch a comedy, talk to someone, do what you love instead.

Repeat as needed.

The more you anchor yourself in the love and fire inside, the less disease, pain, and exterior problems can affect you. Anchoring in love enables detached witnessing: in it, but not of it. Anchoring in the fire helps burn out disease. Remember, the real you is not sick, but getting your body to come back to homeostasis can take time. Practice makes perfect.

MEETING FEAR

With long-haul Covid, I would experience great moments of anxiety, and I would often wake up in the middle of the night with a panic attack or in a tremendous sense of dread and fear. Sometimes I felt like I was losing my mind. This symptom is common among long-haul sufferers.

In my opinion, the only thing to fear is the fear in your mind. Fear is generated in the mind, so it's the mind we must watch. Fear arises when we perceive a threat, whether real or imagined, or carry a false belief that threatens our sense of self: *I'm going to die. I'm worthless. I am a monster. I am losing my mind. I am afraid you will hurt me. I am afraid I am powerless.* The more we focus on fear, the more it clamps down and inhibits our life and actions. This is not to say we aren't experiencing a very real pain, but can we soften our fear and not worry so much about it?

Fear teaches us a lot about ourselves if we can listen to its voice without reaction or attachment. We can stand firm in love and approach each moment as a choice: we can choose fear, or we can choose love.

Whenever you feel fear and pain creeping up, use the Stop, Drop, Walk exercise described above. Slow your breathing, Relax and feel into the center of your heart. Soften and think about the things you love to generate a feeling of love. Ignore the fear that swirls in your mind. The heart does not feel fear, and from here you can choose a positive belief form.

This does not mean you should stand by and let Covid eat your brain. Not at all. Anchor in a place beyond the fear and act from there. In fact, with the love that you generate, you can go into the pain and liberate yourself (and the disease) with fire. We'll discuss this feat in the next chapter. Also check out the Covid Panic Emergency Meditation in appendix 3.

BLESS THE ENEMY

In the first meditation in this chapter, we focused on anchoring on the love in ourselves in the form of a flame. But what if we love the disease? What if we send love out to Covid? To the spike proteins? Can we melt the disease in love?

When I was sick with Lyme disease and at my wit's end, I took myself out to the desert, far from anyone, and sat and prayed for ten days. During that time, I had a profound breakthrough. I realized how much fear I was in. How much anxiety I had about the Lyme taking me over like a monster. But why was I so afraid of a bacteria?

Then I had a breakthrough. What if I loved the Lyme?

A thousand bells went off in my mind. Ding ding ding ding! Yes! Jackpot.

I had heard about disarming a monster by loving it. Jesus said, "Love your enemies" (Matthew 5:44). The Buddhists talk about fierce compassion. Martin Luther King Jr. spoke of meeting hate with love. I knew I had nothing to lose. I imagined Lyme as a baby alien spider, and I held it like a baby and poured all my love out to it. I lovingly cradled *the disease*. I saw it as part of the universe, as a life-form like any other. No matter how terrible its impact on me, it was still part of creation. I kept pouring out love to it and cradling it like an imaginary baby. Surprisingly, I began to feel a sense of compassion for Lyme. For a moment I saw it as an innocent being that had mutated into something distorted, like a fallen angel. I believe even the most hardened criminal still has a human soul beneath the surface, a speck of light somewhere in their heart, a tiny ember of love somewhere behind their walls. I believe that all life has meaning, that all life is sacred, no matter how distorted it may appear to us. I applied this same concept to Covid, and you can, for that matter, with any "disease." When I blessed the Covid enemy, I had a pretty profound experience of the "signature" of Covid and why it was here (see chapter 11). This melting of the disease in love was an important part of my healing from long-haul Covid.

In a sense, I believe loving a disease weakens it, just like someone who practices martial arts will bow to acknowledge the enemy before dispatching them. Loving the enemy does not mean standing by and letting it wreak havoc on your body by any means. Rather, by compassionately ridding yourself of the disease, you are, in a sense, liberating it, as you free it or burn it back to the universe. We can begin to have compassion when we know someone's story or what they have been through. What is Covid's story? What is your story?

I believe nothing can harm the real you when pure love pours out of your heart to the enemy. Make it a practice every day to love every part of creation, even the scary ones. Dark souls and entities exist in the universe, but if you know that they are being harmful or causing an injustice, you can help liberate them by simply blessing them with all your heart. When you unconditionally love all creatures and beings as part of creation, this does not mean that you accept their harm or injustice or don't protect yourself, but rather that you empower them to heal. When you send them unconditional love and pray for their liberation from suffering, you pray for your liberation from suffering. I believe this is what Jesus meant when he said to bless the enemy. So, then, we can pray for the liberation of Covid, helping it melt back into the universe.

⚕ Melting the Disease in Love Meditation

Lie down or sit and make yourself comfortable. Close your eyes. Begin to take some deep breaths. Roll your head gently in circles. Take some deep, slow, wavelike breaths, bringing the air deep into your belly and then rising up to your chest. Full inhalation, full exhalation. Relax and let go with each exhalation.

Continue to breathe slowly and deeply. Now soften your jaw. Soften your eyes. Soften the optic nerve that runs all the way from your eyes back into your brain. Soften your ears and the little ear bones.

Soften the back of your head (the occiput). Soften the juncture where your spine meets your brain. Breathe, relax, let go.

Soften deep in your brain. Imagine that your head is melting downward, like melted butter, sinking and flowing into your heart, bringing your awareness to this center of love. Breathe. Begin to think of the things you love. What do you know you love? Babies, mountains, rivers, birds, a pet . . . Breathe.

Now, once you have generated the feeling of love, imagine the spike proteins, colorful little Tinkertoys holding fast to cells in your body. Don't be afraid. Hold them like little babies. Bring them all into your heart. Cradle them. Bring them to your heart flame. Acknowledge them. Take a deep breath and pour out into them all the love you can muster. Allow all the love of the universe to flow through you in a mighty wave. Call on angels and guides, the white light of a billion suns, the Christ light, for their love to amplify yours. The more love, the better. Take another big breath and again, with a mighty wave of love, flood the "enemy." Flood your entire body. See the little spike proteins in your heart fire popping and transforming into harmless sparks of light that float off to the stars. (Or see them melting into butterflies, or transforming into lights, or whatever works for you.) Increase the frequency, the vibration, within you, becoming a faster light, so that no lower-order energies can harm you ever again. Burn them into a million harmless fragments. Liberate them with your love.

Take another deep breath, and now send that flood of love to your own divine heart, to your own light. Thank yourself, and bow to your heart. Slowly open your eyes.

Option: Instead of meditating on what you love, generate love by loving someone else—a partner or lover, for example. Caress them, adore them, kiss them, hug them, and then, with that feeling of love, call the spike proteins into your heart to be "liberated" in love.

Practice the above meditation as often as you can. It can become the most powerful tool in your medicine kit.

AFFIRMATIONS

When you find yourself having negative or limiting thoughts, try to catch them before you spiral downward. Practice instead the Stop, Drop, Walk exercise and any of the others in this chapter. You will start to feel and notice changes in your beliefs. You will start to let go of worrying and obsessing about your condition so much.

To stay in the "love zone," it is helpful to have affirming statements that you can say out loud or silently to yourself. Try to feel them as you say them. Try singing them. Try using them with the emotional freedom technique (EFT), tapping them in (you can find diagrams of simple EFT points online). Imagine when you say "I am . . ." that you are speaking from the heart, from the place of unconditional love.

Here and at the end of some of the following chapters, I'll offer helpful affirmations to practice, though of course you can make up your own.

Affirmations to Anchor in Love

I am the powerful presence of divine love at all times.

I am the infinite flame of love, knowing no beginning and knowing no end.

I am the loving presence that easily transmutes and melts this disease.

I am always victorious, anchored in divine love.

I am healthy in body and mind.

✺

There is a light that never dies, a flame deep inside,
A place of refuge, a place to hide,
that's always by your side,
A flame that never dies.

4

✦ ✦ ✦

The Fire in the Belly
Protecting and Channeling Inner Vitality

I BELIEVE THAT DEEP IN THE CORE OF OUR BEINGS there is a fire: a spirit fire, the fire of life. It has many names; in other traditions it is called chi, prana, manna, and kundalini. Many cultures have described it as a source of energy and spiritual insight. It's that fire in the gut or core power that motivates us. For our purposes we will call it "the fire in the belly," the fire of existence, that ember that can become like the sun.

In this chapter we focus on building this inner fire.* I believe, when well stoked, this fire will burn out disease, help you face down fear, and keep you alive.

PHYSIOLOGICAL VS. ENERGETIC FIRE

In this chapter we focus on the energetic component of the fire in the belly. But that fire has a physiological aspect as well: our digestive fire. This form of our inner fire is quite literally the fire that helps transform the food we eat into energy.

---

*Building and protecting inner vitality are necessary regardless of your specific circumstances and challenges. Many of the sections in this chapter were drawn from *Liberating Yourself from Lyme,* chapter 3, "The Fire in Your Belly Is the Only Pill You Need."

So much neural tissue lines the digestive tract that some scientists call the gut the second brain (Sonnenburg and Sonnenburg 2015). The neurons of the gut are connected to feeling what is happening in the digestive tract, unlike the neurons in the brain, which organize systemic functions. Gut neurons are more connected to intuition or sensing, giving rise to the expression "trust your gut." It is the fire that calls us to action as the driving force that helps us to create and be dynamic in the world. It is our zest for life, urging us to climb a mountain, rock out, surf great waves, or make passionate love.

On a physiological level, this fire in the belly plays a key role in healthy immune functioning. New research is demonstrating that inflammation and imbalance in the gut may be implicated in many different health issues, including autism, immune dysregulation, schizophrenia, depression, and other related illnesses (Garcia-Gutierrez, Narbad, and Rodríguez 2020).

We know that the Covid virus likes to hit the gut first and knock out the immune army quickly (Ma, Cong, and Zhang 2020). The virus and other pathogenic "bugs" that the virus enables can overwhelm the "good" bacteria in our gut, especially if we have predispositions, deficiencies, or unresolved infections. On top of that, we have to deal with a new intolerance for certain histamine-rich foods. So, healing the gut (see chapter 8) and building our inner fire (the subject of this chapter) become key.

FIRE DAMPENERS

In long Covid, a few crucial questions are: What's causing our immune system to malfunction? What is compromising the ability of our immune system to burn through and liberate the disease? What is dampening our fire? To find out, we may need to look beneath the physical surface.

Suffering and pain from any debilitating and chronic illness is part of the experience, but in addition to genetics and predispositions, there are often unfelt emotional layers beneath that the disease calls to the surface for healing and feeling. There may be outdated patterns and beliefs, unresolved trauma, stagnant relationships, weak boundaries, ancestral karma, or more subliminal psychic pain lurking beneath the disease itself. These conditions can create a sense of powerlessness. Carolyn Myss refers to this in her book *Anatomy of the Spirit,* describing how "the loss of power is the root of all disease" (Myss 1996). This powerful statement may take some warming up to. But it is also the belief of many shamanic traditions and many Eastern systems of medicine that all illness originates in the energy body before manifesting in the physical body.

> *When I check in with myself, I have to acknowledge that I carried Covid to my roommate, and he got quite sick. He was upset with me for months afterward. I remember feeling guilty about it the whole time, and I would say that that guilt weakened my energetic fire and was an energetic factor for Covid developing into long haul.*

In my opinion, if we are fully present in our bodies, grounded and coming from our power or fire, it is not easy for an illness to take hold. Perhaps this is one more reason why some people do not become sick with Covid, have only a mild case, or recover from it quickly, with no long-haul symptoms. Genetics and predisposition play a definite role in the risk for and severity of infection, but it's certainly reasonable to think that the strength of our inner fire—the power of the immune system—plays a part as well. Emotional burdens hamper our inner fire, so addressing them is key to preventing and healing from chronic illness such as long Covid.

Note: This is not to suggest that people with long-haul Covid have made themselves sick, or that everyone who gets sick has an emotional issue. It is both dangerous and unkind to add a layer of guilt and shame to the already stressful situation of suffering. Blaming the sick for their illness is a shadow-side assertion or dark side of the New Age movement. It's nonsense.

It is likewise not helpful for the ill to blame others for their illness or see themselves as victims of circumstances. It is far healthier to take responsibility for the illness and become a force of healing. In other words, by accepting the reality of the condition and looking at what is present and how it can be shifted, we bring the power back into our own hands. As a result we become the creators of our destiny instead of the victims of a dark reality, especially when an illness is chronic. It's also wise to look at the deeper issues of why we may not be getting well. When we begin to move these underlying or energetic blockages, we naturally begin to return to our fire, or life force.

Unfelt Feelings

Chinese medicine teaches that anger and rage are stored in the liver (Kaptchuk 1983). I have no doubt that this is the case; I have felt it many times within my own body. I recall a time when a massage practitioner was doing Chi Net Sang, or internal organ massage, and as she was working on my liver a deep anger and rage overtook me. Fortunately she was able to recognize this, and I went outside to move the old anger without hurting anyone.

Could it be that diseases like Covid and Lyme set up shop in stagnant areas of the body—that is, areas of unfelt feelings? Or that these unfelt feelings dampen the immune system? I, and many others, would say yes. There are many a scientific paper on trauma and the link to autoimmune conditions and chronic diseases (Mock and Arai 2011).

There is an incredible amount of power in the body that can also cause destruction if not properly channeled, like an out-of-control fire. I believe that a tremendous amount of potential energy resides in anger, which can be put to good use if we channel it correctly. If we choose to use that primal energy of anger and rage efficiently, it can become a motivator to fuel the fire for achieving our deepest heart's desires and healing.

I believe fire can quite literally burn out disease, including Covid and any lingering spike proteins. By looking at the emotional aspect of disease and moving any old feelings that might be dampening the immune system, we come one step closer to a more powerful immunity.

During my early journey with Lyme, I was easily swayed by others and was regularly taken advantage of. People described me as spaced out, flaky, vulnerable, and wishy-washy. I often felt as if an unseen force was psychically attacking me, attempting to suck me out of my body, and I was unable to do anything about it. I was panicked by the situation, and my stomach would often churn and be in knots. Partners would often trigger deep feelings, which were quite challenging to deal with, and underneath my symptoms were old feelings of frustration, anger, and rage. A sense of helplessness would creep in, as I would often feel overwhelmed by all that was arising.

A breakthrough came when I stopped blaming others for what I was feeling (or not feeling) and accepted responsibility for my own problems. Ownership is key to the healing process. What is really there beneath the surface?

I gradually began to see that the people I was struggling with were mirroring my subconscious, and I started looking within myself when I was triggered by others, instead of lashing out. I started to pay attention to what was beneath the layers and consciously work on healing. The external patterns finally began to shift as I became aware of old buried pain that had nothing to do with who or what was triggering me. My partner triggering me was a blessing in disguise, as I later learned, an invitation to delve deeper into myself and feel the *unfelt* feelings buried deep within.

Our triggers have the potential to awaken us, to bring us back to full power. A disease like long-haul Covid may be summoning you to become aware and heal old feelings stuck inside your body, deep in the cellular memory.

What would it be like to let go of that which is no longer serving you, embrace forgiveness and gratitude, and access what you truly want in your life? So much of healing is feeling the feelings that never got felt. The immune system responds to this. When we move these old feelings, we reach the power that lies beneath the pain, we connect back with our fire and remove blockages that may be compromising our immune system. At the very least, we check this box and can move on.

Ancestral Feelings, or Epigenetics

What if we go back even further? What if the unfelt feelings of our ancestors are causing the malfunctioning of our immune system? The study of epigenetics says just that: we can inherit the unfelt feelings and traumas of our ancestors, passed on as genetic changes (Nugent, Goldberg, and Uddin 2016). What if we can heal those traumas?

I had a wild intuitive moment about the Neanderthal genetics that appear to increase the severity of Covid in some people. Doing an intuitive meditation, I "felt" into the Neanderthal DNA within me. I held it tenderly and lovingly. What did I feel? I was shocked: that Neanderthal genetic heritage showed me tremendous anger and bitterness. Why? I began to think about it. Didn't Homo sapiens come out of Africa into Europe to find Neanderthals already there? Neanderthals died out around forty thousand years ago. There are a number of theories as to why, but the obvious one is that Homo sapiens won out. The overlap between the two species was only a couple thousand years, and in that time, we took everything from them—including, as we now know, some of their DNA through interbreeding (Ko 2016). Today Neanderthal DNA exists within many of us as just a small piece of our genetic heritage, less than 5 percent of our total DNA. But that 5 percent, I am sure, was not from a pretty thing: rape, or something nonconsensual (I doubt the term even existed then), is the far more likely candidate. Whatever the case, if I were Neanderthal, I would be extremely angry and bitter about the fate of my people. Perhaps those feelings were passed down. Can DNA from that far back still hold unfelt feelings? I would say yes. This is all quite far-fetched, I know, but it offers an example of reasons why our immune systems may be compromised.

Perhaps it's far simpler than it seems; perhaps there are some unresolved, unfelt feelings deep in our genetic makeup that need to be acknowledged and released. So, then, a forgiveness practice becomes key.

✢ Ancestral Forgiveness Meditation

Put on some calming music or nature sounds. Lie down and make yourself comfortable. Close your eyes. Send a grounding cord down from your tailbone to the center of the Earth. This helps to ground you in your body and the Earth. Begin to take some deep breaths. Breathe in, counting to four. Then breathe out, counting to six. Squeeze your whole body, then let go. Relax.

Feel your feet. Relax them. Soften. Breathe.

Feel your head. Relax your jaw as you exhale. Breathe. Relax your eyes; breathe. Relax your ears; breathe. Relax the back of your neck; breathe. Let go of your mind and relax into your physical body. Just breathe.

Imagine that your head is melting downward into your heart, bringing your awareness to this center of love, as if your sensory perception of the world now comes from your heart. Imagine a flame like a candle there.

Begin to think of the things you love. A pet, a partner, a child, trees, the ocean, snowcapped mountains . . . Keep thinking of what you love until you generate the feeling of love. Take a deep breath.

Now take that feeling of love and use it to call up an ancestor or a little bit of DNA you would like to heal. It may be the conqueror or the conquered—whatever is calling for attention the most. Bring that person or fragments of DNA into your heart and cradle them from there, like a mother would hold her baby. Rock them gently. Tell them you love them. Use all your senses to feel into them. Lovingly ask, *What's the matter? What do you need?* Breathe and *listen*. What are they saying? See, taste, smell, hear, feel—use every bit of your sensory perception. Breathe, relax, and listen.

Stay in this place for as long as you like. If your mind wanders, return to the feeling of love by thinking about what you love. Keep pouring out all your love to your ancestor DNA. Then ask for forgiveness. Ask to be forgiven for anything you or your ancestors may have done. Feel what arises in you. Let it go. Let it wash out. Pour out more love. Say silently, *I'm so sorry, I love you. Please forgive me/us.*

Take a big breath and again pour out to that ancestor or DNA as much unconditional love as you can. Now forgive them for anything that was done to you. Say silently, in that loving cradle, *I forgive you.* Let it go. Breathe. Pour out as much love as you can muster. *I forgive you.*

Now once again think about the places, people, pets, and things you do love. Pour all of that love and golden energy into your own heart. Place your hands upon your heart and forgive yourself.

Optional: As an alternative, modify this meditation to be sung or danced. Put on some good music and do a dance of forgiveness.

Forgiveness lies at the core of healing. Self-forgiveness is at the peak of what I call the "triangle of forgiveness"—the other two points being forgiveness of others and asking for forgiveness. It's the hardest but by far the most important. Forgiveness cannot be forced; it can take days, months, and sometimes years to finally let go. Though it takes time, if you practice every day, like a steady drip, one day the bucket will overflow. Your immune system responds to forgiveness. Consider some sort of offering, retribution, or restoration for the "sins" of the past. Is there something you can do to make peace with or for your ancestors? Perhaps make an altar, plant a garden in someone's honor, or perform an act of reconciliation. Check out the book *Braiding Sweetgrass,* by botanist Robin Wall Kimmerer, who talks about offerings to ancestors as well as offerings to the Earth for the unprecedented destruction of flora and fauna we are currently witnessing.

BUILDING FIRE

After we have worked with forgiveness, we want to reclaim our power, to access the tiger within, to get the fire good and hot, to burn through disease. Breathwork, qigong, martial arts, yoga, lovemaking, spending time in nature, or doing anything that gets your fire stoked is essential for building fire. Passive sweating, hot saunas, infrared saunas, hot tubs, hot baths, fats, and fire foods (such as cayenne, garlic, and ginger; see chapter 8) all help tremendously, but the best thing you can do is to feed the energetic fire in your belly. Even just thinking about some activity you love to do can help; if you are lying in a hospital bed, you can start just with feeling that little spark in your core.

Physical Exercise

Exercise stimulates the production of epinephrine (a.k.a. adrenaline) in the body, which, in turn, triggers the production of monocytes (Geraghty, Hann, and Kurtev 2019). In other words, these white blood cells become more active, but that's exactly what we don't want for Covid long-haulers because amped-up monocytes exacerbate symptoms. Instead, we want to calm this overactive part of the immune system. So, we must do gentle exercises at first, gradually titrating up as we feel better. I remember going for a long run in an attempt to build my cardiovascular strength; I thought it might help my battle with long Covid. The next day I had a massive headache, and I felt miserable for days. Lesson learned.

As I got better I was able to very gradually increase my activity levels until I was eventually able to exercise without any kickback. You will have to find your own threshold and ramp up slowly.

Some gentle exercises that won't get your heart rate up too high include walking, yoga, gentle bouncing on a trampoline (which helps move lymph), lifting weights (if you take extra time between sets), qigong, and tai chi. When you begin to improve, try jogging, maybe just around the block to start, as this can get your lymph moving.

Meditations to Build Fire

Many breathwork modalities offer powerful methods for stoking our inner flame and building immunity. I present two of my favorites below. There are others, including the popular Wim Hof Method. I also suggest the yoga practice called nauli, or abdominal churning, with your breath held; this increases carbon dioxide levels in the blood, which stimulates the vagus nerve to calm the nervous system, and increases the fire in the belly. You can explore these techniques online.

Another effective exercise is one I developed called the Fire Love Loop; the name refers to the way in which it combines the use of inner fire and love to liberate disease from the body. See appendix 2 for details.

Whichever methods you choose, I suggest practicing fire-building breathwork twice a day, in the morning before eating and again in the afternoon.

𐩒 Breath of Fire Exercise

Find a comfortable place to sit or stand. Hold your arms up above your head, pointing your thumbs to the sky. Begin a series of rapid exhalations and inhalations, emphasizing the exhalations. Do thirty. Then take a big breath and hold it for at least thirty seconds, and longer if possible. Exhale forcefully, like a dragon. Repeat three times or more.

𐩒 Fire Stick Meditation

Lie down or sit and make yourself comfortable. Close your eyes. Begin to take some deep breaths. Roll your head gently in circles. Take some deep, slow, wavelike breaths, bringing the air deep into your belly and then rising up to your chest. Full inhalation, full exhalation. Relax and let go with each exhalation.

Continue to breathe slowly and deeply. Now soften your jaw. Soften your eyes. Soften the optic nerve that runs all the way from your eyes back into your brain. Soften your ears and the little ear bones.

Soften the back of your head (the occiput). Soften the juncture where your spine meets your brain. Breathe, relax, let go.

Soften deep in your brain. Imagine that your head is melting down-ward, like melted butter, sinking and flowing into your belly, as if the very seat of "you" existed in your gut. Breathe.

Take in a big breath and, on the exhalation, relax and soften your gut. Place your awareness just below your belly button and back, in toward the spine. Now, breathing calmly and slowly, imagine you are going to build a fire there, the way our ancestors did with a fire stick. Imagine taking that stick between your hands and placing the point in that center spot below your belly button, just at the front of your spine. Imagine a little bit of tinder there. Breathe deeply and calmly. Begin to twirl the stick back and forth, slowly but firmly. Stay focused; stay relaxed. Spin the stick faster and faster, digging in. Stay focused on that "hot spot." Feel it beginning to warm up. Feel the heat. Faster and faster you spin, staying steady, focused, and firm. Now you can see some smoke rising up. Keep spinning the stick until you see an ember, a little spark, glowing in the tinder. Feel the heat. Now pause, and imagine bending down to blow on the ember. Breathe in and blow out, gently, with your lips pursed, just like you would nurse an ember into life; steady focused air.

See the fire spark to life. Now it is a small flame. Put some kindling on it. Throw some anger on it; think of some injustice that makes you angry, and use it as fuel for your fire. Try to feel the heat of the fire. When the fire is big enough, place a log on it. Now it's nice and hot, a good steady flame with hot embers and coals forming. Stay there.

Now imagine that this fire is like a magnet, like the sun and its gravity, drawing oxygen and energy toward it. Relax the rest of your body. Breathe deeply. Imagine the fire is magnetizing any disease, the spike proteins, the dark confused cells, misformed cells, viruses and bacteria that do not belong inside you . . . See all the harmful bugs and bad cells being inexplicably drawn to your fire. As they reach the fire, see them pop, spark, and burst into flames. Bless them and roast them. Imagine them transforming to something greater. See spike proteins turn to harmless sparks, see "bugs" turn to butterflies, see bad cells turn to little sprinklings of peace. Liberate the disease. Melt it back into the universe.

When you are ready, take a big breath, thank yourself, thank the proteins and bugs and bad cells for what you have learned, open your eyes, and be done.

Practice this exercise as much as you can, along with the Melting the Disease in Love meditation in chapter 4 and the Fire Love Loop exercise in appendix 2. When you combine love and fire in this way, you are in a sense blessing the enemy, then sending its ass back to kingdom come.

Choosing to Heal

I believe that deep within your body there exists not only the desire but also the wisdom to heal yourself. Your body knows the way. The knowledge exists within your cells. It lives in your immune system within the red and white blood cells that know how to fight illness. At some point you will undoubtedly be able to access your body's healing force to heal yourself, though it might just take some time to remove the blockages. I encourage you to be patient with yourself and your healing process. It takes time and patience and a commitment to choose to heal. Have faith and trust that the fire in your belly can burn through disease. Imagine you are running a marathon and need to stay focused and disciplined.

One of the most awakened spiritual teachers was Thich Nhat Hanh, a Vietnamese monk who witnessed horrific atrocities during the war in Vietnam. He was forced to flee his homeland and live in exile for more than forty years because of his peaceful resistance to the violence on both sides. He suffered severe trauma, yet he used that energy to fuel his inner fire and generate such a well of compassion, healing, and forgiveness that his teachings have spread across the world.

Perhaps there may be a particular political or environmental issue that sparks a sense of justice in you, that makes you stamp your feet and want to do something about it. Try to feel that fire; feel your passion. What is it that stokes you? Who or what is it that you love and is worth standing up for? Start small if you need to; perhaps it's your pet or a tree. Take notice, and keep stoking, for, I believe, it is that stoke that can burn out disease.

Affirmations to Build Your Inner Fire

I am the infinite flame of love, easily burning through any disease.

I am the fiery presence that easily transmutes and melts this disease back to God.

I melt the disease in the mighty fire of my core.

I am powerful beyond measure.

By the mighty flame in me, I command you, nomads, be gone!

❦

There is a vitality, a life force, a quickening that is translated through you into action, and there is only one of you in all time, this expression is unique, and if you block it, it will never exist through any other medium; and be lost. The world will not have it. It is not your business to determine how good it is, not how it compares with other expression. It is your business to keep it yours clearly and directly, to keep the channel open.

MARTHA GRAHAM

5

◆ ◆ ◆

Calming the Storm
Natural Relief for Chronic Inflammation

LONG-HAUL COVID IS A DISEASE OF CHRONIC INFLAMMATION, both neural and vascular. The lingering spike proteins or viral debris, autoantibodies, and corresponding damage appear to be the main culprits, as we explored in chapter 1. This chronic inflammation can set up a kind of PTSD reaction in the limbic system and amygdala, the area of the brain that stores trauma. We get stuck in a loop, caught in an immune malfunction, a signaling of faulty messages over and over again. In essence, a constant fire rages in our brain, and we need to calm it down. In this chapter we explore techniques and meditations to reset and help calm the overreactive immune system. We'll look at medicines and supplements in chapter 9.

REST

Rest is your most important ally in recovering from long Covid. Our immune system works best while we're resting, and that is also when our glymphatic system takes out the trash (see chapter 7; Besedovsky, Lange, and Born 2012). Try to get as much rest and relaxation as you can get—more than you think you would need. Take naps or just lie down often. If you're able, take a sabbatical or go on a retreat. Even finding moments throughout the day where you can just lie down for twenty minutes can help calm the storm and relieve imflammation.

It may be hard for your family and friends to understand why you are still sick and needing so much rest, and that can be frustrating. Just remember—and remind them—many people have been dealing with long-haul Covid symptoms for more than two years now. The better you take care of yourself at the outset, the sooner you'll find relief.

> I intuitively "heard" the words rest, chill, and relax so many times that resting became the number one priority on my daily to-do list.

MUSIC

Studies have shown that listening to calming music can aid the limbic system, and classical music can help build new neural connections (Helsingin 2015). Listen to relaxing music or soothing nature sounds often. Make a playlist of your favorite calming tracks, and look for music designed specifically for healing, utilizing frequencies and tones for maximum benefit. (You can find many of them online.)

> I found the sounds of gently flowing water to be the best for calming me down. These sounds helped me imagine the inflammation washing out of my body.

WATER

What puts out the fire? Water. This element will be one of your best allies. Drink as much water as you can daily to calm inflammation and flush the lymph system. Get good springwater if you can. And try drinking ice water. Ice helps calm inflammation and also stimulates the vagus nerve (see below). You can also ice your body or even just your head. Try an ice bath or, if you can find a source, cryotherapy. Ice, baby, ice! Get in cold water, too: rivers, lakes, oceans, baths, pools, or cold showers.

⚕ *Ice Mountain Meditation*

Find a quiet space and put on some gentle water sounds. Or find a quiet spot by moving water—a burbling brook, rushing river, lapping waves. Make yourself comfortable. Close your eyes. Begin to take some deep breaths. Breathe in, counting to four. Then breathe out, counting to six. Squeeze your whole body, then let go. Relax. Continue to breathe deeply.

Imagine a cool, calm, deep mountaintop lake. Icy peaks surround it. Everthing here is cooling, icy, calm. Breathe into the stillness.

Calm and soften your brain. Bring the still, cool pool into your brain. Imagine the water gently washing through, calming and cooling your brain and any inflammation found there.

Now imagine a gentle stream of cool, calm water washing down from your brain and through your body, clearing out any debris, bringing it down through you and out.

Then imagine a cobalt blue light pouring through your brain and body, continuing this peaceful calming energy and clearing your energy field.

BALANCING THE AUTONOMIC NERVOUS SYSTEM

The autonomic nervous system is made up of two parts: the sympathetic and parasympathetic. The sympathetic nervous system activates the fight-or-flight response in the face of a threat or perceived danger, and the parasympathetic nervous system restores the body to a state of calm (Waxenbaum, Reddy, and Varacallo 2022). The word *sympathetic* is really the wrong word; it's more like *frightened* nervous system. Imagine the word *parasympathetic* as having a parachute, lightly and gently bringing you down. So for cases of long Covid, where the body is in a state of chronic inflammation and stress, we want to activate the parasympathetic nervous system and calm the sympathetic nervous system.

Boosting Carbon Dioxide Levels

As we saw in chapter 1, blood-gas balance can be disrupted in long-haulers. In particular, carbon dioxide levels can be low. It turns out that carbon dioxide helps calm the nervous system and feelings of anxiety, activates the parasympathetic nervous system, and has anti-inflammatory effects (Otterbein et al. 2000; Wolpe 1987). It also increases blood pH—and one indicator of Covid severity is low blood pH (Patel et al. 2022; Kieninger et al. 2021).

> I "saw" many times that there is a gas imbalance with long-haul Covid, and I often had images of the gas (carbon dioxide) coming off a freshly opened bottle of soda. I also had images of breathing into ballons or paper bags and rebreathing that CO_2.

So, try drinking carbonated (sparkling) water and nonsugar sodas and practice visualizing the effervescence and bubbles calming the fire of inflammation within. And use the breathwork techniques described below to boost carbon dioxide levels in your blood.

Calming the Limbic System and Retraining the Amygdala

In long Covid, the sympathetic nervous system gets stuck in fight-or-flight mode, leaving the immune system overstimulated and overreactive. This "PTSD" loop has its origins in the limbic system.

The limbic system is located in the center of our brain, at the base. This part of our brain mediates our behavioral and emotional responses, especially those behaviors we need for survival: feeding, reproduction and caring for our young, and fight-or-flight responses. The limbic system is made up of the following structures:

- Hippocampus—involved in the formation of new memories, learning, and emotions
- Amygdala—involved with emotions and traumautic memories
- Thalamus—acting as the body's information relay station

- Hypothalamus—responsible for the production of important hormones and the regulation of thirst, hunger, mood, etc.
- Basal ganglia—responsible for reward processing, habit formation, movement, and learning

The amygdala is a little almond-shaped structure at the base of the brain. When a person senses danger, the amygdala sounds the alarm and the hypothalamus activates the sympathetic nervous system. The adrenal glands respond by pumping adrenaline into the bloodstream, which triggers the release of blood sugar and fats—giving the body a surge of energy (Rajmohan and Mohandas 2007).

Release of the stress hormone cortisol from the hypothalamus and pituitary can drive the amygdala to stay in fight-or-flight mode. Cortisol levels have been found to be significantly lower in long-haul, causing weakness, fatigue, and low blood pressure (Klein et al. 2021).

In a study of post-Covid brain scans, the pituitary, hippocampus, and amygdala were found to be chronically inflamed or of a larger volume than normal (Tu et al. 2021). This inflammation can cause the myriad hormonal and glandular issues we see in long-haulers.

The inflammation of the hippocampus in long-haulers can result in dysregulation of brain regions essential for fine motor function, learning, memory, and emotional responses, as well as loss of neurogenesis and hormonal disorders, psychiatric disorders, and other issues (Klein et al. 2021).

Inflammation of the brain stem can also result in dysregulation of the hormone serotonin and can create psychological and mood imbalances (Boldrini, Canoll, and Klein 2021).

So, calming the limbic system; reducing inflammation in the hippocampus; regulating cortisol and other hormones, such as serotonin; and retraining the amygdala through neuroplasticity techniques like the Gupta program become high priorities for long-haulers. The following breathwork techniques can help.

Breathwork

For our purposes, we want breathwork techniques that can calm the nervous system and shift us into the parasympathetic state. The long, slow breathing techniques that increase carbon dioxide levels have shown the greatest benefit for calming the system (Russo, Santarelli, and O'Rourke 2017). Following are some of the ones I found helpful.

⚘ Calming or Box Breath

This kind of breathwork is great for both calming your nervous system and getting to sleep. All the breathing is done through the nose. In the morning, breathe in for a count of four, then exhale for a count of six. At night, before going to bed, inhale for a count of four, hold for a count of four, then exhale for a count of four.

Alternatively, you can try Dr. Andrew Weil's 4-7-8 version: inhale for a count of four, hold for a count of seven, and exhale for a count of eight. My favorite is inhaling for a count of six, then pursing my lips and exhaling with a *shhhh* sound for a count of ten.

⚘ Buteyko Breathing

Buteyko breathing was developed by Ukranian doctor Konstantin Buteyko to help his chronically ill patients. It is similar to box breathing, but the emphasis is on increasing carbon dioxide levels to relieve conditions like asthma and anxiety. The slow, relaxed breathing and increased carbon dioxide also activate the parasympathetic nervous system. Buteyko breathing also builds nasal nitric oxide, which helps increase the amount of oxygen the blood can absorb.

Inhale through your nose as slowly as possible, then exhale as slowly as possible (for longer than the inhalation period), until you feel air hunger. To boost the effectiveness, then hold your breath for thirty to sixty seconds. So, it might look like this: inhale for a count of six, exhale for a count of eight, then hold your breath for thiry seconds.

❧ Wim Hof Method

This ever-popular method was developed by Dutch extreme athlete Wim Hof, who claims that it reduces inflammation and the pro-inflammatory cytokine response. Deep breathing increases oxygen saturation in the blood, while holding your breath increases carbon dioxide levels.

A typical practice is this: Take thirty slow, deep, powerful breaths, bringing the breath up from the belly to the chest. After the last breath, exhale and hold your breath for one to two minutes or longer. Repeat for a total of three cycles.

Wim Hof likes to combine this breathing practice with ice baths, which has a further anti-inflammatory effect, as discussed earlier.

I found myself doing Wim Hof breathing in the morning, as it was more invigorating, and the other breathing techniques like Butyeko afterward or when I was having symptoms. After doing one of the breathing practices, I'd place an ice pack on the back of my neck, at the base of the brain.

You have to find what works for you, and there are many more breathwork techniques awaiting discovery. My own technique, the Fire Love Loop exercise (see appendix 2), can also be effective.

VAGAL NERVE STIMULATION

The vagus nerve, the longest nerve in the body, runs from the medulla at the base of the brain all the way to the colon. This nerve supplies parasympathetic fibers to all the organs, and that is what we want: more parasympathetic actions to calm long Covid's chronic fight-or-flight response (Breit et al. 2018).

Polyvagal theory, introduced by psychiatrist Stephen Porges in 1994, describes the autonomic nervous system as having three subdivisions that relate to social behavior and connection. First is the dorsal vagal system, a part of the parasympathetic nervous system, which enables us to shut down or freeze when a situation of danger feels uncontrollable and we are overwhelmed. Second is the fight-or-flight system, mediated by the sympathetic nervous system. Third is the ventral vagal system, another part of the parasympathetic nervous system, which governs social engagement (Porges 2009).

Increasing your vagal tone activates the parasympathetic nervous system, and having higher vagal tone means that your body can relax more quickly after stress. So, we want to stimulate the vagus nerve to help calm the body, release trauma, and interrupt the overreactive fight-or-flight response that is typical of long Covid.

Vagal nerve stimulation consists of applying electrical stimulation to the vagus nerve. Cold exposure also stimulates the vagus nerve, as does deep and slow breathing that increases CO_2, singing, humming and chanting, gargling, probiotics, chewing gum, exercise, massage, and laughing (Howland 2014).

There are also some simple exercises for stimulating the vagal nerve. You can find many of them online. Here's one of my favorites.

⚗ Vagal Nerve Stimulation Exercise

Sit in a chair. With your right hand, reach up over your head, bend your elbow, and place your right hand over your left ear. Use this hand to gently pull your head to the right in a gentle stretch. Then, moving your eyes but not your head, look up to the left. Hold this position for thirty to sixty seconds. Breathe normally. Then switch sides and repeat.

NEUROPLASTICITY RETRAINING AND NEUROGENESIS

As we know, Covid and other diseases and trauma can injure the brain, activating the limbic system and keeping us in a constant state of stress and dysregulation. But the brain has neuroplasticity—the ability to rewire itself and heal—in response to new experiences and information. Neuroplasticity is defined as the ability of the brain to form and reorganize the synaptic connections between neurons, creating new pathways. Neurogenesis is the ability to grow new neurons. We now know that the brain has a tremendous capacity for repair and renewal if it is given the right tools to do so.

Neural pathways are like grooves in a record, guiding our mental processes along known patterns. Sometimes those patterns are not beneficial, though, and we get stuck in a rut worrying about our body, feeling anxious, having negative thoughts, and so on—including the experience of the sympathetic fight-or-flight response triggered by long Covid. Neuroplasticity training helps create new grooves or patterns, giving us a powerful tool for improving mental and physical health.

A number of programs, like Dynamic Neural Retraining (DNRS), the Gupta Program, Brain Gym, emotional freedom technique (EFT), eye movement desensitization and reprocessing (EMDR), and many others, have specific practices and exercises to help rewire the brain, calm the limbic system, and resolve trauma (Shaffer 2016). Also, any kind of crossing-the-body activities, like crossing your hands to play piano or cross crawl exercises, for example, can help new neural connections to form, as can learning new skills and having new experiences. The Stop, Drop, Walk exercise in chapter 3 is another good way to set new neural patterns. The New Groove exercises on page 57 is yet another.

I tried many practices to help calm my nervous system and found the Gupta Program, created by Ashok Gupta, to be particularly helpful. Researcher Ashok Gupta developed his program after suffering for years with chronic fatigue syndrome. This program, like other neuroplasticity trainings, focuses on rewiring the brain and getting us out of the limbic loop through a series of meditations and a seven-step process of developing new healthy patterns. When you're sick with a chronic illness like long Covid, much of your time can be spent worrying about what's wrong and obsessing over your symptoms. I stopped worrying about my symptoms after going through the Gupta Program, and I noticed improvement in my mental and physical symptoms, too.

⚘ New Groove Exercises

From my practice as a bodyworker and somatic therapist I have found that doing figure-eight movements with the body helps rewire nerve function and erase old faulty patterns.

Find a space where you can move around freely. Stand in a slight crouch with your legs spread widely, as if you were mounted on a horse. Hold your arms out in front of you, elbows slightly bent, palms down. Now swing your arms in toward each other and let them cross over, right arm on top, rotating your palms to face upward as you do so. Then swing them back out again, turning your palms to face down again. Repeat, now letting the left arm be on top. Continue this wave-like figure-eight movement, swinging in one continous movement. When you're ready, slowly start bending, so that you are swinging your arms lower and lower as you go, and swing them from the top to the bottom of your body and then back up. Do three sets.

If you are familiar with the chakras, you can do one set of arm swings at the level of each chakra, visualizing your swinging movements cleansing each chakra as you go.

Another great practice is to simply place your index finger just on the edge of your peripheral vision. Look at it with both eyes. Then move it to a new location, just on the edge of your vision, and look at it. Move the finger all around your peripheral vision and repeat.

DISSOCIATIVE MEDICINES

Many long-haulers have had success using dissociative and psychedelic medicines to support their recovery. These include ayahuasca, iboga, ketamine, psychedelic mushrooms, LSD, San Pedro cactus, and more.

These medicines can help us break out of the limbic loop and calm the nervous system by dissociation, disarming the hyperreactiveness of the immune system (Feder et al. 2020). Microdosing (or macrodosing, if the situation calls for it) these medicines can also improve mood, reduce anxiety, and help with immunomodulation (Szabo 2015). Many studies have shown the effectiveness of these medicines for chronic illness; we will explore them more fully in chapter 10. The homeopathic versions of these medicines may be of benefit, too. Be advised of the legal status of these medicines, if you go this route, and be sure to work with an experienced shaman, healer, or psychotherapist.

GRATITUDE

Cultivating gratitude can go a long way in changing not only your mind-set but also your biochemistry (Fox 2017). When we are ill we tend to focus on what's wrong, but what if we focused on what was good? For example, if your left arm is in pain, find a part of your body that is not. Is your right arm in pain? If not, can you be grateful for it? Can you find gratitude for the things that *do* work in your body? For the ones you don't even have to think about?

⚕ *Gratitude Cover Meditation*

Lie down or sit and make yourself comfortable. Close your eyes. Take three deep breaths. Relax. Now begin to scan your body, and notice where there is pain. Take notice and acknowledge the pain. Just leave it for now.

Take a big breath. Now find a part of your body that is not in pain, something that works just fine. Feel into that place with your senses. What does it feel like? Can you describe what a good feeling or a good part is like?

Take a big breath. Now bring in the feeling of being grateful for that part that is not in pain, that is working as it should. Hug it and kiss it and give it more love, and be so thankful it works so well. *Thank you, thank you, I am so grateful.* Now find that gratitude for your whole body. You exist because of this body. Though it may struggle, it keeps you alive. Give it love, and be so thankful it has worked all this time for you. *Thank you, thank you, I am so grateful.*

Big breath. Now take that feeling of love and gratitude and use it to cover the pain. Smear that gratitude/good feeling right over the pain. Push that feeling of gratitude right into it. Visualize a golden light oozing into every cell there. Tell this part you love it, you need it, and you know it can heal. *I know you can heal, I love you, thank you, thank you.* Visualize that part of your body working properly and with no pain whatsoever.

When you are ready, close the meditation with a prayer and bow to your heart.

We often get so caught up in what's wrong that we forget about what's right. Focusing on pain and what's wrong can get us stuck in a loop. So, forget about it for now and go focus your attention elsewhere. Read a book, do a crossword puzzle, watch a comedy, talk to someone, and so on.

Affirmations

I am grateful for the love I have in my life.

I am regulated and calm, normalizing all functions in my body.

I lovingly bring my limbic system back to normal.

I am healthy, relaxed, open, and healed now.

I am rewired for optimum health.

6

✦ ✦ ✦

Immune Commune

Techniques for Energetic and Physical Immunity

WHAT IS IMMUNITY? Webster's dictionary defines it as the capability of multicellular organisms to resist harmful microorganisms, and also the capacity to recognize and tolerate whatever belongs to the self, and to recognize and reject what is foreign (non-self).

On the physical level, then, the immune system is like a protective army. This army has billions of cells—soldiers, special forces, support staff, generals, and all *sorts* of munitions—at your service. It even has spies and rogue traitors. Sometimes the army attacks the self. This is autoimmunity. Sometimes our army becomes weak or important aspects don't function correctly. Sometimes that's because the immune system is hampered by, among other things, genetics, emotions, or exposure to toxins like certain molds, chemicals, radiation, food allergens, pathogens such as bacteria and viruses, heavy metals, and so on.

On the energetic level, the ability to reject what is foreign and recognize what is self can be disrupted by emotional issues. For example, what if we don't love or trust the self? What does that say to the immune system?

When you're faced with long Covid, the first questions to ask are:

What factors might be hampering my immunity? How do I find out what I need to heal? To remove those dampeners of immunity? To make sure my immune system is functioning optimally?

Even if your immune system is working just fine, supporting that immunity is key for recovery.* We'll break this chapter into two parts, first approaching energetic immunity, then looking at the nitty-gritty of physical immunity.

ENERGETIC IMMUNITY

Consider that the immune system also has an energetic component, and it may be greatly influenced by our emotions, thoughts, self-love, stress, trauma, ancestral trauma, karma, and so on. We might say that energetic immunity in its ideal state is love, or being in alignment with love and the self. This self-love allows a protection of boundaries, a "standing firm against those that would seek to harm thee."

Our immune armies are stronger when we love them, when we support them, when we want to protect the castle. I call this love and fire, or self-love and boundaries. Consider that self-love may go a long way in building immunity. This does not mean that you won't ever get sick; it just means that you will fare better and recover more quickly because your immune system is working more efficiently.

Consider that self-love may involve forgiveness and gratitude. Consider that emotional blocks may hamper the flow of energy and the health of the gut, where most of the immune system resides.

Self-Love
What does self-love mean to you? How do you feel about yourself? Don't like or trust yourself? Don't like a part of your body? If you have an unconscious loop going that says, "I don't love myself," what does

---

*In fact, the information in this chapter is relevant regardless of the disease or circumstances you're up against. Many of the sections in this chapter were drawn from *Liberating Yourself from Lyme,* chapter 5, "Building Immunity."

that say to your immune system? Why should your powerful army go out and protect you if you yourself don't care about you? And what does it mean to have autoimmunity? Could that imply self-sabotage? Consider that the simple act of self-love and self-care strengthens your immune army.

Consider that self-love might mean simply giving yourself the space to be who you are. Perhaps taking yourself to a place of acceptance. Doing the things you love to do. Being around the things you know you love. No obligations involved. Ask yourself how you could be more in alignment with what you love. Consider that being out of alignment with what you love can hinder your immune system.

What would it feel like to forgive yourself, or begin to forgive yourself, for the misgivings and mistakes of the past? Can you forgive yourself for getting Covid? Consider that self-forgiveness is at the heart of health.

Consider that the cure is already in your body, that your body knows what it needs to heal, that your immune system is an incredibly intelligent, adaptive, sensitive, powerful community. How can you support the immune system in doing its task? How can you get the immune system, your powerful internal army, in tip-top shape?

Forgiveness

I remember lying in bed, sick with Covid, feeling so helpless. I was so upset with myself for being careless and not taking the coronavirus more seriously. I was upset at whoever it was that gave it to me, and even more upset and guilty that I had given it to a housemate. I worked on forgiving the person who had given it to me as well as seeking forgiveness from the person I had given it to. But I was still pissed. Then I had a thought: I had forgotten to forgive myself. Over the years I have come to understand that self-forgiveness is really at the heart of healing. As I began to forgive myself, and consider the lessons I had learned, I noticed a sensation of letting go.

"Shit happens, and I did what I could. No use in beating myself up about it. Just be the lesson and move on," I thought.

I could *feel* how forgiving myself strengthened not just my mind-set but my actual immune function. I began to feel better, emotionally and physically. And that makes sense; if I am having negative thoughts and feelings about myself, how can my immune system not feel the same? Can my immune system function at 100 percent if I don't love myself? Likely not.

Forgiveness is at the heart of healing. Forgiveness is the key to awakening the heart. Releasing old grief and anger is paramount for healing. Forgiving ourselves and those who have harmed us as well as asking forgiveness from those we have injured or hurt in some way can help us return to a natural state of love. Try to make this effort a daily practice; it may take time, perhaps lifetimes, but you can discipline yourself like an athlete who is training for a race. This discipline empowers us to take responsibility for what is, instead of blaming anyone outside ourselves. We are choosing our power to heal through forgiveness. Self-love charges our immunity. To love, accept, cherish, and nurture ourselves, just as we are, is, I believe, a reclamation of our power.

Inner Fire

What in us is dampening our inner fire, defender of our boundaries? What is inhibiting our ability to keep invaders out of the castle? What's keeping our inner flame from burning bright?

We discussed the factors that dampen our inner fire in chapter 4. Consider them carefully. Who or what is draining you? Who or what are you draining? Holding healthy boundaries is a form of self-love. Stronger boundaries—stronger fire—strengthens the immune army.

⚕ Immune Boost Meditation

Lie down or sit and make yourself comfortable. Close your eyes. Take three deep breaths, bringing these slow, deep breaths down into your belly. Relax.

Focus your attention on your heart center. Think about what makes you happy: the experiences, people, or things that you love. Generate a feeling of love in your heart. What does love feel like?

Take a few more slow, deep breaths, breathing into your heart center. As you inhale, think or say, *I am love.* As you exhale, think or say, *I love.* Generate as much love as you can in your heart. Keep breathing deeply.

Now exhale, and with that exhalation, send that love out through your whole body. Hold yourself like a baby, cradling your body with as much tenderness and compassion as you can. Adore yourself; imagine yourself as a baby, and hold and love that baby. Be open to anything that may arise. Breathe.

Now begin to imagine your immune system as an army with millions of specialized cells that are ready for action. See all the new baby cells in your gut, your bone marrow, your pancreas, or wherever suits you. Now send this army of cells the same love that you just generated in your heart. They need your support, so flood them with as much pure, golden light as you can. Flood your gut and the marrow of your bones with this love. Flood the thymus, pituitary, and pineal glands. Flood the lymph, blood, and anywhere else in your body where immune cells are standing by, awaiting your guidance, with this love. Hold them all like valiant warriors, deep within the love of your heart. Give them all the strength and courage they need. You are the general of this army. Tell them about the sneaky enemies, spike landmines, and rogue soldiers on this journey to healing. Tell your soldiers they are more powerful than the invaders. Using your mind's eye, show your immune army pictures of spike proteins and viral particles. Show them the enemy. Then, once you have blessed your soldiers, it's time for them to go out there and liberate the enemy.

Now call on your inner fierceness to face the spike proteins that are trying to hide from your immune system. Then drop down into your gut and see or feel the hot red fire that lives there, the flame of your immunity and sigil of your invincible army. Instruct your immune army to march out with swords and fire to melt, eat, burn, and liberate the invaders that would seek to harm your body. Say to yourself, *I am always victorious; I melt and transform these nomads back to the presence of divine love,* or *In the name of the mighty God presence within my being, nomads release!* or whatever feels authentic to you. Permit yourself to have boundaries. Feel the victory within your body.

Take some deep breaths again and imagine sealing your body with a protective field that cannot ever be penetrated. Love is the victor.

Practiced daily, this energetic exercise can bring tremendous results, especially when used in conjunction with your medicines. Many times, I have looked into my body and seen how the spike proteins have entered the immune cells and are trying to fool the immune army, keeping themselves disguised. We have to keep telling our armies that they are smarter until they know it. Stand as strong as you can in this truth until every cell of your body believes it.

The Fire Love Loop exercise in appendix 2 can also be used for boosting the immune system.

Negative Thoughtforms

I believe the energetics of disease feeds on fear and negative thought-forms. What is a negative thoughtform? It is anything that is not essentially based on love. For example, a partner breaks up with you, and you form the thought, "I am not worthy, something is wrong with me." Then guilt and fear creep into your psyche. As we've seen time and again, negative feelings and negative self-image have negative effects on our biological function. And disease feeds on this process.

I believe that some negative thoughtforms are crystallizations of trauma and unfelt feelings. Consider how your thoughts might relate to old wounds. As you acknowledge old unfelt feelings, your thoughts and beliefs may naturally change, and vice versa. See chapter 4 for further exploration.

Attitudes and Beliefs

Just as important as physically supporting the body is emotionally supporting the body. The moment you choose to heal and decide to get well no matter what, you are on your way. It's essential to believe that you can kick long Covid. You can coach yourself or even get a life coach or someone who can help you with positive thinking. Being positive can be hard when you're going through such a challenging disease. Try imagining that the world is counting on you, and you will be amazed by what you can do. Take on the mind-set of a long-distance runner: you are running a marathon, not a sprint. Stay focused on the goal and pace yourself. Practice your daily affirmations and whatever else you need to do to stay on the path. Be open to all the possibilities your intuition might reveal. Call on the magic—it's out there! We live in a universe of infinite possibilities and probabilities. Healing is not just one of those possibilities but a probability. Your body wants to heal, and it's your remembering and choosing that can help it do its job. Make it a daily statement: "I choose to heal." Visualize yourself totally healthy.

We all have a tendency to focus on what's wrong. For example, we may put a lot of energy into thinking about Covid—how much we hate it and the pain it creates and how we are going to kill it. As a result, we neglect the healthy parts of ourselves. We often say things like "I am sick" or "I have long-haul Covid." But are *you* really sick? Is the deepest part of you truly sick? You can go ahead and believe that, but consider that the deepest part of you may not be sick at all. Your pain is real, but perhaps your body is going through some type of initiation. What part of your body works just fine? Why not focus on what is healthy and spread that around? When we believe we are sick, it can take longer to heal. By changing our beliefs, we can change our bodies, and even the pain.

⚕ Healthy Feeling Meditation

Lie down or sit and make yourself comfortable. Close your eyes. Begin to take some deep breaths. Roll your head gently in circles. Take some deep, slow, wavelike breaths, bringing the air deep into your belly. Full inhalation, full exhalation. Relax and let go with each exhalation.

Continue to breathe slowly and deeply. Now soften your jaw. Soften your eyes. Soften the optic nerve that runs all the way from your eyes back into your brain. Soften your ears and the little ear bones.

Soften the back of your head (the occiput). Soften the juncture where your spine meets your brain. Breathe, relax, let go.

Soften deep in your brain. Imagine that your head is melting downward, like melted butter, sinking and flowing into your belly, as if the very seat of "you" existed in your gut. What does that feel like? Soft and relaxed. See all the thoughts and worries dropping into the earth. Breathe.

Now find a place in your body that is healthy and not in pain—your white blood cells, perhaps, or the little toe on your right foot, or your nose, or deep in the center of your heart. Or remember an activity that you love to do when you are feeling healthy—surfing, skiing, making passionate love, climbing a mountain, or laughing. What does that health—in your body or in your experience—feel like? Capture that feeling of good health. Bring it into your heart. Focus on it. Rest and breathe into that place. Allow your thoughts to be pulled down into your heart. See how they may change.

Now take that feeling of good health and begin to spread it around your body. Spread it far and wide; spread that health to all parts and points in your body and energy field. Let it wash and melt over the pain and thoughts that have plagued you. Begin to say slowly, *I am strong, I am whole, I am healthy, I am powerful.* Remember what health feels like. Feel it and begin to believe it. Let the feeling permeate your whole being.

Open your eyes when you are ready.

Monitor your beliefs about yourself and your health, and watch out for negative thinking. Whose voice is talking? Is it a voice of fear or love? You get to choose. Remember that your body believes every idea you think, so choosing positive thoughts can help you heal. Many methods and techniques for reprogramming and repatterning can be of help, such as emotional freedom technique (EFT), neuroplasticity programs like the Gupta Program, or eye movement desensitization and reprocessing (EMDR).

One technique I found very helpful is this: When you notice you are thinking negative or self-defeating thoughts about yourself or someone else, pull those thoughts into your heart. Imagine they are little tendrils of energy (which they are) and pull those little crystallized negative thoughts down into your heart. Hold them in love, feel them melt there, and see what new positive thoughts arise.

Touch

Touch and lovemaking are some of the most important ways to boost your immune system, and they're fun, too. Merely brushing your own body or touching another brings smiles and love to our hearts. It also increases serotonin levels in our body, making the immune system happy (Ellingsen et al. 2015). Choose to love and care for those around you. It is essential to hold and touch each other. A pet is a wonderful companion—another being to form a healthy bond with and to give and receive unconditional love. Loving and caressing our bodies can help, too. Consider reaching out to those who are worse off than you: they are aching for love.

Ultimately the immune system functions as a conduit for healing the entire being. Let yourself love and be loved, and do what you love.

A Free Flow of Energy

What is health? This is an important question to ask ourselves. I believe that health, at its core, is *a free flow of energy.* This was a phrase that popped into my head one day. Imagine an electrical line that conducts energy quickly along power lines. If there is a blockage, the energy cannot move. We know the entire universe has an electrical component, as do our bodies. How can we keep that free flow of energy moving? Tai chi and qigong practices work with this concept. Below is a simple exercise based on a qigong exercise.

☃ Free Flow of Energy Exercise

Stand in an area (preferably outside or in a park) with enough room to extend your arms. Bend your knees slightly, as if you were riding a horse. Slowly inhale and lift your arms from your side, palms up, scooping them straight up over your head. Let the palms turn down and bring your arms down in front of you while you slowly exhale. Repeat. Imagine a waterfall or river cascading down through your crown and washing through you as your arms descend during the exhalation. Imagine that water flowing through you and into the earth, cleaning out emotions, Covid, and any "trash."

This is a simple exercise to do when you feel tired or drained. It is a form of energetic hygiene that will keep your system healthy and flowing, rather than stuck and constricted. If you are bedridden, simply imagine a gentle stream pouring in at your crown and out through your tailbone with the rise and fall of your breath.

Make Love and Fire Your Main Medicines

It becomes apparent that increasing love and inner fire (boundaries) is paramount for immune support. This becomes the foundation. Keep this as your main focus. Look to build from the inside first, rather than relying on the external only. Then you can focus on all the foods, exercises, remedies, and other external components that support immunity.

Get Out of the Way

We have a lot of "intervening" practices to help you get better, but there is also a place of trust, of getting out of the way of the innate healing process. In other words, don't get too focused on trying to "fix" the immune system. Just sending yourself love goes a long way.

Affirmations to Build Energetic Immunity

I am the powerful presence of infinite love, calming and harmonizing my immune system.

I command my beautiful army to regulate and stand down.

I am home. Come home, cells who have run away, I love you.

I harm not myself.

I harmonize my immune system and upgrade it with more love and strength.

I am powerful beyond measure.

PHYSICAL IMMUNITY

We have explored what might be dampening our energetic immunity, but what then might be dampening our physical immunity? And what can we do to help it? Remember that with long-haul Covid, it's not so much about building your immune system as it is about calming it and making it smarter and more efficient. The immune system can learn—in fact, that's its job—and it can learn to heal your body from this virus.

The immune system is such an incredible, adaptive, vast array of cells and systems that scientists are still working out the details. It's like its own universe. For simplicity's sake, immune cells can be categorized as lymphocytes (T cells, B cells, and NK cells), neutrophils, and monocytes/macrophages. These are all types of white blood cells. The major proteins of the immune system are predominantly signaling proteins (a.k.a. cytokines), antibodies, and complement proteins. It is usually the monocytes and neutrophils that are involved in autoimmune disorders like what we have seen with long Covid (Navegantes et al. 2017).

Autoimmune Retraining

Some researchers theorize that long Covid is a disease of autoimmunity, where the immune system attacks the very antibodies that it sent to fight the virus, as discussed in chapter 1. It's as if this new form of virus has confused our immune system, sending its armies into chaos. How then can we smarten or reeducate our immune system? How can we teach it to better distinguish between the spike proteins and its own cells and antibodies?

During my intuitive meditations, I clearly heard the word malfunction *in relation to my immune system, and on numerous occasions I had an image of a switchboard with crossed wires.*

. . . .

Immune Malfunction

As discussed previously, with long Covid the immune system does get its wires crossed, so to speak, over the spike proteins. The immune system is in overdrive. It's like the gas pedal is on the floor but the car is not in gear. We have this mélange of dysfunction: auto-immune or idioantibodies, T cell (CD57) exhaustion, immune check-point inhibitor malfunction, hormonal disruption, and much more. So then calming, modulating, regulating, and retraining the immune system becomes very important. This is done through a variety of drugs like CCR5 inhibitors, immune checkpoint inhibitors, low-dose nal-trexone, medicinal mushrooms (reishi, chaga, turkey tail, etc.), herbs like ashwaganda, neuroplasticity retraining techniques, breathwork, homeopathics, dissociative drugs like ketamine, and much more. We discuss remedies in chapter 9

. . . .

Some concrete physiological methods for retraining the immune system are being investigated. One is to continually reintroduce fragments of the offending culprit to help educate immune cells in a kind of immunotherapy. In a study conducted by the University of Birmingham (2020), for example, scientists presented the immune system with repeated doses of a fragment of cells—in this case proteins of the myelin sheath—that white blood cells were attacking. Repeated exposure to these fragments helped to desensitize the immune system and stopped its attacks on those proteins. This is similar to the process of allergy desensitization, where you introduce tiny amounts of the offending culprit. This model could help explain why some long-haulers have benefited from the vaccine; reintroducing the offending culprit (the spike protein) may trigger the immune cells to go take another look and "teach" the immune system to distinguish between the offender and the body's own cells. Studies are under way to verify this. Studies have also shown that vaccinated individuals are less likely to develop long Covid in the first place (Venkatesan 2022).

Another way to retrain the immune system is to receive information from an immune system that has already healed from Covid. Monoclonal antibody therapy, where lab-made antibodies help educate the immune system, fits this model (Gupta et al. 2021). Currently researchers are developing specific monoclonal antibodies to block the Covid-triggered autoantibodies (Chen et al. 2021). Keep an eye out for new developments in this arena.

> In my intuitive meditations, I would often "see" images of cows and milk bottles. My wife even put her hand on my aching brain one time and said, "I see a cow." Then one day I "saw" an image of a bunch of milk bottles and another bottle of milk that could be used for injections. "Ahh, colostrum!" I thought. Turns out colostrum has an incredible amount of immunoglobulins that can clear out foreign particles and modulate the immune system (plus it helped me with headaches). But injectable? Yes, this is called intravenous immunoglobulin (IVIg) therapy—these immunoglobulins are derived from antibodies or plasma from humans—and it has been found helpful for Covid and "smartening" the immune system (Kolahchi et al. 2021).

But what about the autoantibodies themselves? Can we reeducate them? Or get them to stop? To stand down? Many doctors use steroids and other immune suppressants to do just this, as well as a technique called plasmapheresis (which basically entails removing the offending autoantibodies). Medicinal mushrooms like reishi and chaga also come in handy here. We'll discuss these techniques and medcines in chapter 9. For now, perhaps we can disarm these rogue antibodies with visualization.

⚕ Rogue Soldier Meditation

Lie down or sit and make yourself comfortable. Close your eyes. Begin to take some deep breaths, bringing them down into your belly. Now focus your energy on your heart center. Start thinking about and feeling into what you love: experiences, people, places, or things. Generate that feeling of love in your heart. Take a few more slow, deep breaths.

Now visualize the immune cells that have gone rogue in your body, the autoantibodies. See the confused ones. See them as old warriors who have done a tremendous service, fighting valiantly. Gather them all up and hold them like little babies. Bring them into your love, into your heart. Call them in from all parts of the body. Pour out to them as much love as you can. Thank them for their service. Honor them. Tell them you love them and instruct them, lovingly but firmly, to calm down and to go. *Thank you so much for your work. It's time to let go now, it's time to come home, it's time to allow yourself to retire. It's safe to let go and relax, let go and die, it's all okay, the enemy is not coming back to life. We love you, we need you, come home.* Take a deep breath and pour out more love to them.

Then call out to the universe (or God or whatever feels appropriate to you) and ask for an upgrade to your immune system. Ask for a rewiring. Imagine a river of golden light flooding through your body, washing out the garbage, the old cells and trash. Ask for a DNA download: *Divine DNA download now!* Relax, and visualize a proper rewiring taking place, as if a computer upgrade is downloading for a few minutes.

Now imagine holding the new baby white blood cells. The new ones popping out from the bones and places they are made. Send them all your love and instruct them to be valiant. They are not to attack the body anymore or the viral trash, like the old soldiers did. The old ones are dying. That's okay. Let them die. Hold the entire immune system in your heart. Send a wave of love through your immune system and the new cells and trust that now it will recognize any spike proteins and either break them down or not touch them.

When you are ready, take a big breath and thank yourself and your immune system. Allow yourself to be in awe of the intelligent and beautiful immune system.

By holding the "bad" cells in love, you are asking them to transform, to recalibrate, to "come home" and let go of killing the wrong things. Your love can make them stronger and wiser. But you must be firm and in command. You must be the general of your army, wise and compassionate, but fierce. I encourage you to take the above meditation, put on some good music, and sing and dance to it. Dance with your immune system, bring joy to yourself, bring the soldiers back home. Bring out the new smarter little white blood cells. Allow the cycle of life and death to take its natural course within you. Trust, surrender, pray.

The Stressors

In addition to genetics, which we explored in chapter 1, there are a number of immune stressors to assess and minimize. Clearly poor diet, lack of exercise, lifestyle stress, exposure to molds and toxins like pesticides and heavy metals, exposure to radiation and electromagnetic frequencies (EMF), trauma, and vitamin and mineral imbalances all play a part in the immune system's overall health. See chapter 8 for a discussion of diet; below, we'll talk about some of the other stressors that are particularly key in the struggle to heal from long-haul Covid (or any disease).

Lifestyle Stress

So much has been written about stress and its negative effects on the immune system that we won't get into it here. Where can you trim out stress? What relationships, work, or living situations are no longer serving you? Where can you calm down, simplify, and relax? Where can you find romance, walks in nature, or meditation time? Though huge life changes are likely not possible when you are ill, trim the stress where you can. What stressors in your life can you get rid of or walk away from? What initiators of joy and peace can you have more of? Make a list of what stresses you out, and see what you can realistically minimize. Then try rest, meditation, breathwork, gratitude practices, retreats, and sabbaticals to support your well-being.

Electromagnetic Field Overload

You may need to minimize your exposure to electromagnetic fields (EMFs) to continue on your healing path. With long Covid, your energetic field and central nervous system are already compromised. The additional strain of dealing with EMFs can pose another obstacle to your healing. It is essential to remove yourself from high-frequency fields for your immune system to function optimally. The elderly, children, and those who are ill are much more susceptible to these frequencies than are healthy adults (Ng et al. 2012).

There are new peer-reviewed scientific studies showing the connection between long-term exposure to EMFs (from wireless technology, electrical outlets and towers, and 5G and a vast array of new frequencies) and an increase in long-haul Covid symptoms. Such EMF exposure can result in the depletion of substances like glutathione, exacerbation of heart issues, disturbance of biochemical regulators in the blood, and dysregulation of the immune system (Rubik and Brown 2021).

Pay attention to any signals your body may be giving you in response to an EMF overload. You will need to minimize your screen time as well. Most of us have a threshold. Find yours.

How close are you to a cell phone tower? Cell phones run on microwave frequencies, and there is some evidence that this may be harmful (Moskowitz 2018). Where is your head in relation to power sources in your home when you sleep? Sources include power strips, outlets, and computers. Is the power line hookup to your house near your bedroom? Is the wireless transmitter for your internet on at all times? You may want to consider getting an Ethernet router for your computer, as it has a far lower impact than wireless (Wi-Fi) from an EMF perspective. A separate mouse and keyboard can also help minimize computer EMF exposure.

Try intentionally grounding your energy by taking walks in nature, exercising, bathing, or swimming (especially in salt water) to deal with the strong electromagnetic fields. Many essences and herbs can both shield us from and ground this electromagnetic energy. Yarrow is a particularly important plant that shields the body from electromagnetic radiation (Kaminski and Katz 1994). There are also many EMF blockers on the market, including pendants that can be worn around your neck.

Mold Exposure

As mentioned previously, when the immune system is compromised, other pathogens that are normally kept in check, like mold, can gain a foothold. Mold can seriously complicate the Covid presentation and has been found in high levels in some severe Covid-19 patients (Rabagliati et al. 2021).

Molds like the common *Aspergillus* can create aflatoxin, a toxic substance that permeates the air we breathe. Aflatoxin can get into the lungs and impair the body's ability to heal by compromising the immune system (Khlangwiset, Shephard, and Wu 2011); it can also trigger other conditions like MCAS (Kritas et al. 2018).

Mold in closets and bathrooms, under carpets, in corners or windowsills, in attics and cellars, and even outside can inhibit proper immune system function. Exposure to these moldy hot spots must be avoided or minimized for the immune system to perform optimally. If you live in a house with a mold problem, I highly recommend considering relocation to a sunny spot. Both your health and well-being depend on it. You can have a specialist come to your home and test for mold.

If you can't remove yourself from mold at the moment, here are some insights I have gained. You can work on mopping up mold in the body with products like zeolites, chlorella, and the probiotic *Saccharomyces boulardii*. Curiously enough, tobacco smoke helps kill mold, especially when the mold is in the lungs (Parmenter and Uhrenholdt 1976). If you are dealing with long-haul Covid in a place with mold issues, consider taking an occasional puff of organic, additive-free tobacco every so often, or blow tobacco smoke around moldy areas. Although regular smoking certainly isn't healthy, the occasional use of tobacco (two or three puffs of organic tobacco once a week) could outweigh the negatives. The little hairs in your lungs called cilia are damaged by tobacco smoke. However, they grow back stronger, similar to a person who lifts weights and then rests to give muscles time to rebuild (Tashkin and Murray 2009; UK Essays 2013). Tobacco is also an important antiviral, as we explore later in the book (Shang et al. 2016).

Another option is agave, or century plant, whose juice can reduce aflatoxin levels in the body (Rosas-Taraco et al. 2011). In addition, agave has very high levels of saponins, which I believe are an important medicine for long Covid, as we will discuss in chapter 9 (Yang et al. 2006).

Urine tests revealed that my own mold levels were high, even though I was living in a very sunny, mold-free environment. As I did with Lyme disease, when I was living in a moldy house, with long-haul Covid I kept "seeing" both agave and tobacco. I had previously discovered that tobacco can inhibit the growth of mold in the body, but with long-haul there seemed to be another connection: nicotine. It turns out that nicotine, the potent chemical found in tobacco, may inhibit the Covid-19 virus and reduce the cytokine storm (Korzeniowska et al. 2021). I found many a forum on nicotine and long-haul Covid; many sufferers tried nicotine patches and claimed that they interfered with the spike proteins and ACE-2 receptors. More study remains to be seen, but intuitively I believe that tobacco—when used in small amounts—is a powerful ally for long Covid.

Body Chemistry Imbalances

Researchers are discovering that Covid-19 can cause biochemical imbalances in the body. It may be that as inflammation affects the brain and glands, secretions of hormones like dopamine, cortisol, serotonin, acetylcholine, and and other chemical compounds can fall out of balance.

For example, the attack on the immune system leads to a sudden loss of insulin-producing beta cells, causing acute hyperglycemia, or high blood sugar. Many long-haulers become at risk for diabetes or pre-diabetes (Barrett et al. 2022).

The pituitary gland often becomes inflamed with long-haulers. Because it regulates other glands and hormones (in fact, it's sometimes called the master gland), this inflammation can throw all sorts of functions out of whack, including testosterone and estrogen levels (Bordes 2021).

In addition to the systemic inflammation, long-haulers can experience biological abnormalities including redox imbalance (weakened antioxidants), an impaired ability to generate adenosine triphosphate, and a general hypometabolic state (Paul et al. 2021). Electrolyte imbalances also occur, with low serum concentrations of sodium, potassium, and calcium (Lippi, South, and Henry 2020).

Elevated biomarkers in Covid-19 patients include D-dimer (may indicate a blood clotting condition), N-terminal pro-B-type natriuretic peptide (NT-proBNP; may indicate an increased risk of mortality from heart problems), C-reactive protein, ferritin (stores iron), procalcitonin (from infections), and IL-6 and IL-10 (cytokines) (Lopez-Leon et al. 2021).

Patients with severe Covid have also been found to have low levels of uric acid (Dufour et al. 2021). Low uric acid levels have been associated with neurological issues like Alzheimer's, optic neuritis, multiple sclerosis, and Parkinson's disease. (You can increase uric acid levels by taking zinc and/or inosine supplements and by eating animal products and organ meats and foods high in purines, like fish.)

On top of this, repeated physical and emotional stress from the illness is a major trigger for persistent inflammation in the body, which can also affect the brain and shrink the hippocampus, inflame the pituitary, and therefore affect both our biochemistry and our emotions. Stress can also affect levels of cortisol, which can affect our mood. Eventually, these changes can cause symptoms of depression and anxiety.

In a newer study, long Covid patients were found to have low levels of cortisol, which is normally found in high levels with those under stress. This is likely again the result of inflammation of the pituitary gland, which regulates this and other hormones.

> While I was sick with long-haul Covid, I did a ton of bloodwork and came back with the following imbalances: low CD8/57, low FSH and low testosterone, low uric acid, high glucose levels (prediabetic), high cholesterol, low cortisol, high C4a, high TNF-alpha and IL-10, and high CCR5. This was all new, apparently arising from Covid-19, and again mostly a result of pituitary inflammation.

Support the Immune System

Healing Your Gut: Your Composter

Safeguarding the health of the gut is probably the most critical step in overcoming any pathogens. Many studies and much research point to an unhealthy gut as a prime issue in many diseases and conditions, including chronic fatigue syndrome, autism, obesity, and a host of others (Mulle, Sharp, and Cubells 2013).

We now know that 80 percent of our immune system resides in the gut (Wu and Wu 2012). New studies are demonstrating the gut/brain connection as well through the vagus nerve. When our gut is out of whack, this can directly influence the brain, and vice versa (Carabotti et al. 2015). With Covid, the inflammation in the brain is directly related to the inflammation in the gut, and it becomes paramount to get the bacterial gut fire in top shape to fight off the virus and other bugs.

A vast array of bacteria and enzymes that live in our intestines not only help break down food but also serve to halt invading, harmful bacteria or pathogens. When we are in good health, most of these bacteria are incredibly beneficial. They are found in high amounts in raw fermented foods and raw dairy, such as colostrum and yogurt. A healthy gut can adequately digest and nourish the body with essential vitamins and minerals. When our gut is leaky, due to bad food choices, toxins, pathogens, unresolved emotional issues, or genetic predispositions, it becomes much harder to digest foods. A breached gut wall barrier leaves us more susceptible to pathogenic bacteria and parasites. A condition called GAPS (gut and psychology syndrome) can result from chronic inflammation in the gut caused by eating foods, such as grains and complex carbohydrates, that don't digest properly. GAPS is implicated in conditions such as autism and attention deficit disorder (Campbell-McBride 2004). Repairing the gut and strengthening the immune system become of utmost importance as part of cultivating the fire in the belly, which is a powerful ally in healing.

The gut lining itself becomes important to heal. Aloe vera and L-glutamine may help with that. Various dietary protocols, too, can be helpful. Most studies show that eliminating gluten and other grains can be helpful in restoring the gut lining, and for this reason, some long-haulers choose a ketogenic diet, with high fats and very few grains. Then again, other long-haulers choose to eliminate fats to decrease systemic inflammation (Fritsche 2015). I found a high-fat ketogenic diet worked best for my body.

Together, the microorganisms that live on and in us—bacteria, viruses, fungi—make up our microbiome. In a healthy state, these microorganisms exist in a self-supporting balance. Dysbiosis—that is, disruption of the microbiome's balance—is associated with severe Covid and may play a role in long Covid (Chen and Vitetta 2021; Hirayama et al. 2021). For this reason, it may be helpful to offer support to the beneficial bacteria that populate the gut. We can do this with prebiotics, meaning the food or fiber that these beneficial bacteria eat and use to proliferate. Prebiotics include foods and herbs like chicory, dandelion, garlic, onions, asparagus, and more—such as agave inulin (Thomas et al. 2021). We can also incorporate into our diet probiotics, meaning foods that actually contain these beneficial bacteria. They include yogurt, buttermilk, raw milk, kefir, fermented vegetables, and more (Singh et al. 2017). You can also find many probiotic supplement formulas. One particular probiotic, *Bacillus subtilis,* among others appears to be effective at inhibiting Covid-19 (Alam et al. 2021).

. . . .

The Good, the Bad, and the Ugly

In my meditations focusing on the gut I would often hear the word *buttermilk*. Buttermilk is high in bifidobacteria. I would also "see" *aspirin* and, curiously, *Coca-Cola*. I had always heard that Coke can help an upset tummy—and, of course, the opposite, that it is "rot gut"—but then I did a little research.

Researchers have found that in long-haul Covid, specific gut bacteria—both "good guys" and "bad guys"—get out of whack. A 2022 study found decreases in twenty-eight types of gut bacteria and increases in pathogenic ones (Liu et al. 2022). Bifidobacteria, Collinsella, and Ruminococcus are some of the good guys that

have been found to be low in many long-haulers (Bozkurt and Quigley 2020). A gut microbiome analysis can help in supplementing the missing good guys. This can be of great benefit since researchers have found different bugs depending on different symptom presentations. In one study researchers found that treating the gut to Lactobacillus probiotics combined with inulin from chicory root could help with acute and long-term Covid symptoms (Thomas et al. 2021). Butyrate is another supplement that many long-haulers say helps restore balance. Bad guys that flare up include species of streptococcus and clostridium (Liu et al. 2022). Antibiotics like amoxicillin and clindamycin may be used to knock them back.* And guess what else may kill them? Aspirin and coke—the ugly!

Many studies have shown that aspirin and other NSAIDS can disrupt the gut microbiome in a negative way. However, there are also studies showing that aspirin can effectivly lower levels of harmful bacteria, such as strectococcus, as well as biofilms of such bacteria (Veloso et al. 2015). As for Coke, it turns out that it does indeed have an antimicrobial effect—on both pathogenic and beneficial bacteria (Dağ et al. 2015). Coke can also act as a kind of detergent because it contains citric and phosphoric acids (see chapter 7). There is no good science to back the idea that Coke may benefit gut flora, but I believe there's something to it. Perhaps try drinking a Coke now and then and see how you feel.

---

*In addition, parasites such as threadworms and roundworms that were being held in check may need to be knocked out. A parasite cleanse with herbs such as cloves, black walnut, and wormwood may be in order, or antiparasitics like mebendazole may be needed.

. . . .

Unfortunately, many people with long-haul Covid develop a mast cell response and a newfound sensitivity to foods high in histamine. So high-histamine foods like dairy products and ferments may not work for some. We'll explore diets and foods for long Covid in detail in chapter 8.

I found that low-histamine probiotic supplements with bifidobacteria and Bacillus subtilis, homeostatic soil organisms (HSO), colostrum, buttermilk, kefir, a little yogurt, and later a little kimchi or a splash of apple cider vinegar worked well for me. I found cow-derived colostrum was the best for my body, but goat colostrum also works well for many people. I also found that colostrum in pill or liquid form would help bring down a headache.

For more information on restoring the gut, see *The Body Ecology Diet,* by Donna Gates.

Food and Herbs

Many foods and herbs help support the immune system. Since everyone responds differently to the same foods and herbs, a good naturopath or herbalist can be of great help here. The essential foods for long Covid are those that best build fire in your belly and nourish your brain, especially the fats and oils. See chapter 8 for an in-depth discussion on the best diet and foods for long-haulers.

Among the most important herbs for modulating and regulating the immune system are the medicinal mushrooms, such as turkey tail, chaga, lion's mane, and reishi. These mushrooms help "smarten" and rewire the immune system and have been used for thousands of years in Chinese medicine (Guggenheim, Wright, and Zwickey 2014). I believe they are very important for healing long-haul Covid. We discuss them further in chapter 9.

Urine Therapy for Immune Support

When I was taking antibiotics in the hospital years ago when I had Lyme disease, I had a clear vision of peeing into a cup, and I thought, *Oh, no! Drink my pee? You have to be kidding!* Then I did some research. Yogis and many health care practitioners recommend drinking midstream morning urine when your body is ill (van der Kroon 1996). Urea (in urine) has also been found to be helpful for

low sodium in the blood, as is common with long Covid (Decaux et al. 2014). I again had an intuitive hit to try it with long-haul Covid.

My "impression" of how it works is as follows: Because our body is mostly water, and I believe that water carries memory (Emoto 2001), we can assume our urine holds an imprint or memory as well. For example, you can taste whatever has been added to water quite easily, like lemon or fluoride or the fresh taste of a mountain spring. If this is true, we can expect this on an energetic or subtle level.

Because the spike protein hides, the immune system may have a hard time recognizing it to make antibodies (Zhang et al. 2021). This makes it challenging for your immune response to fight it properly. Covid fools the immune system, which gets stuck in a catch-up game with the disease and may even end up attacking the body itself in an autoimmune overreaction. When we take a medicine, we may flush some of the viral trash and broken spike proteins, which are then carried out in the blood and liver to be excreted from the body and appear in the urine. These dead spike proteins can "imprint" in the water or blood of our body. As we drink our urine or water impression and put it back into our bodies, I believe it becomes a self-regulating mechanism. In other words, our body and immune system filter what's coming in, which helps the immune system to recognize the dead spike protein in the urine and creates proper antibodies for it. The urine acts as a homeopathic, boosting the immune system to recognize it or any other infections we may have.

Drinking urine can also help increase our levels of uric acid, which, as we have seen, can be low in long-haulers and can be an indicator of severe Covid (Dufour et al. 2021).

Drink about one-half cup taken midstream from the morning's first urine. Much more information and studies can be found about this age-old practice on the internet.

Medicines

There are many remedies for boosting the immune system, but as we've discussed, with long Covid, it's more about smartening, regulating, modulating, and calming the immune system. Ramping up white blood cells may not be helpful, as they get stronger and just attack the self. So some medicines may work against us and, as I found out, even cause a histamine response.

Herbal medicines that fall into the helpful immune-regulating category are the medicinal mushrooms (and the psychedelic ones), ashwagandha, tulsi, garlic, turmeric, aloe vera, shilajit, and many others (Mahima et al. 2012).

Western pharmaceuticals like steroids (or steroid-like plants), low-dose naltrexone, fluvoxamine, and others can help calm an overreactive immune system (Bolton, Chapman, and Van Marwijk 2020). Please see chapter 9 for more information.

Homeopathics can also be beneficial here. Homeopathic versions of the psychedelics that can calm the brain, and the reptile remedies like Crotalus (rattlesnake venom) can calm the limbic system (Hutchinson 2016). We explore this more in chapter 9.

Vaccine

Long-haul Covid support organizations like Survivor Corps have many reports that the vaccine abated or even completely knocked out long-haul symptoms. It is unclear why the vaccine may help, but it appears that reintroducing the spike protein may jump-start the immune system in recognizing the lingering spike proteins, or perhaps it "distracts" the immune system by creating new antibodies, taking the stress off the autoantibodies. One recent study found that with three exposures to the spike protein (whether through Covid infection or the vaccine), the body develops a robust response to Covid, as well as antibodies that bind to the spike protein (Koerber et al. 2022).

However, the vaccine itself carries some risk of toxicity (see chapter 7), and in rare cases the vaccine can cause long-haul symptoms (see chapter 1). It's a bit of an odds game, and what's right for you may not be right for someone else. This is where you have to trust your gut.

Naps

Our immune system is most efficient during rest (Besedovsky, Lange, and Born 2012). With long-haul Covid, or any disease, it is important to get rest, whether it's a two-hour afternoon nap or twenty-minute resting moments throughout the day. Because Covid can get into the brain and inflame the pineal and pituitary glands, it's often impossible to sleep, as many people with long-haul Covid will tell you. I found that doing yoga or the Breath of Fire exercise (page 44) for about twenty minutes helped me to rest. Box Breath (page 53) is also helpful. Herbs such as valerian or CBD oil can help, as can magnesium.

If you need to take a Western medicine like Ambien to sleep, by all means occasionally do so; just don't let it become a bad habit. I found that if I took a twenty-minute rest during the day when I felt fatigue coming on, I would feel just as recharged as if I had taken a two-hour nap. You don't even need to fall asleep: just lie down, breathe, and let go. Naps are a great way to recharge your battery, but not everyone can sleep during the day, which is why I suggest resting. Rest as much as you can during the recovery period.

7

◆ ◆ ◆

Taking Out the Trash

Methods for Drainage and Detoxification

OVER THE COURSE OF DEALING WITH LONG-HAUL COVID, one of the most consistent images I keep "seeing" was trash inside my brain—dumps, dirty bathrooms, sewage with flies, clogged drains, dirty water, broken toilets, and on. Then I would have images of soaps and cleaners—Ajax, Windex, bars of soap, detergents, dish soap, bubbles, and so on. I even had a dream where I was gargling with soap. Clearly my brain wanted scrubbing to wash out all the garbage. What do soap and detergents do? They break down proteins. Are there proteins we want to break down? Why yes, there are—spike proteins.

Symptom-wise, the sides of my neck and back of my head were always extremely painful and achy. These are the sites of lymphatic ducts draining the brain. Everything always seemed backed up and painful to the touch. It makes sense that if we are dealing with the rotting spike proteins and the dead cells that the autoantibodies are creating, we are going to have very backed-up lymphatic and glymphatic system, like the drain got clogged because of an overload of waste. Keeping this area moving becomes key.

THE LYMPHATIC SYSTEM

The lymphatic system is a network of tissues and organs that help rid the body of toxins, waste, and other unwanted materials. The primary function of the lymphatic system is to transport lymph, a fluid containing infection-fighting white blood cells, throughout the body. The lymph system has no natural pump; lymph is moved by the pressure created by the body's movements, breathing, and muscle contractions. In long-haulers, the cervical and occipital lymph ducts at the base and sides of neck are often swollen and inflamed, thus causing chronic aching at the back of the neck (Distinguin et al. 2021).

THE GLYMPHATIC SYSTEM

Like the lymphatic system, the glymphatic system is a network of vessels that clears waste—specifically from the central nervous system (CNS) and the brain, and mostly during sleep. As with the lymphatic system, the glymphatic system gets backed up with the "trash" of the coronavirus, causing swelling and improper draining (Wostyn 2021).

METHODS FOR MOVING LYMPHATIC AND GLYMPHATIC FLUID

Keeping lymphatic and glymphatic fluid flowing is paramount to detoxifying the body. As these systems have no natural pump, we have to manually help them move with exercise, massage, and other processes. A good hands-on osteopathic doctor, craniosacral practitioner, acupuncturist, or lymphatic massage specialist can help.

Massage
You can find many lymphatic self-massage techniques online, and there are many practitioners who specialize in lymphatic drainage and massage such as effleurage. This type of massage tends to be very gentle, assisting the body in sweeping the lymph. Here is a simple self-massage technique.

⚕ *Lymphatic Self-Massage*

Make sure you are comfortable while doing the massage. You can try a seated, standing, or lying-down position. Use a light pressure and keep your hands soft and relaxed. The pressure of your hands on your skin should be just enough to gently stretch the skin as far as it naturally goes, and then release it. If you can feel your muscles underneath your fingers, then you are pressing too hard. Use the flats of your hands instead of your fingertips. This allows more contact with the skin to stimulate the lymph vessels.

Gently and slowly run your hands down the sides and back of your neck, from your head down to just below your clavicles, gently stretching your skin, then releasing it. Repeat fifty times. Then pause with your hands on your ribs, just below the clavicles, and gently lift your elbows up and down, as if you were slowly flapping your wings. Flap three times. Repeat.

Deep Breathing

Deep breathing not only helps relax the nervous system but also moves lymph through the respiratory contractions, allowing for drainage.

⚕ *Lymph Breath*

Breathe in through your nose, slowly and deeply, for a count of six, letting your stomach and chest expand like a wave. Breathe out slowly through pursed lips for a count of ten, letting your stomach flatten. As you are inhaling, visualize the back and sides of your neck expanding, bringing oxygen to this area. Repeat five times. Take a short rest between each breath so you do not get dizzy.

See also the breathing exercises in chapter 5.

Exercise

As many with long-haul Covid have discovered, exercise, especially cardio, can make symptoms worse. So be careful with exercise; find your limits and listen to your body. Non-cardio exercise worked fine for me, and I was able to ramp it up as I became better.

For moving lymph, any kind of bouncing in place or on a trampoline is helpful, as is yoga, headstands, and lifting weights. Walking and short jogs can help as well. These exercises act as a manual pump; the action of flexing and contracting the muscles helps the lymph move. As you get better, try jumping rope or running.

Dancing is not only a great way to get some exercise and move lymph but also a powerful way to return to your joy and lift your spirits. So put on some music and bounce away.

⁂ Lymph Swing

Standing in place, swing your arms up over your head and then back down. As your arms come up, let your heels come up off the ground; as your arms come down, let your heels come back down to the ground. Repeat as a fluid motion for a few minutes.

⁂ Head Cradle

Lie on your back and place your thumbs behind your ears, across the mastoid bone, as if you were cradling your head. Slowly move your head from left to right with your hands. This helps "pump" the lymph.

Skin Brushing

The skin is our largest organ of elimination. Brushing your skin daily promotes detoxification by stimulating the lymphatic system. You can lightly dry-brush your body before showering, or you can brush while bathing in a hot bath. You can also use tools, like the ridged crystal used in gua sha, to brush along lymphatic channels of the neck.

Herbs for Lymphatic Drainage

Herbs including cleavers, echinacea, licorice, ocotillo, red root (ceanothus), yellow dock, and more, including many from traditional Chinese medicine (Peng et al. 2020), can help move lymph. These can be taken as tinctures.

Rest

The glymphatic system drains when we sleep or rest (Jessen et al. 2015), which gives us yet another reason why rest is important for recovery from long-haul Covid. Additionaly, the supplement phosphatidylserine has been found to help the glymphatic system move waste while we sleep (Lind 2021).

Acupuncture and Cupping

Both acupuncture and cupping (placing heated cups on the body) can help move stagnant lymph and blood.

BODY DETOXIFICATION

A tremendous amount has been written about toxins and detoxification. Research indicates that the increasing levels of heavy metals, petrochemicals, radiation, xenoestrogens, and chemical pesticide residues in our environment are affecting our bodies and dampening our immune systems (Singh et al. 2017). With the rise in cancer and autoimmune disease, it is difficult to deny the connection to these toxins.*

With long-haul Covid, where the lymph and glymphatic systems are constantly backing up with waste, weekly or biweekly detoxification of the entire body becomes important. You can undertake a complete detoxification protocol all at once, though I tried to pick certain days where I backed off on some medicines and just focused on a small detox for the day. Water becomes your most important ally here, so drink plenty of it daily.

There are many herbs and supplements that help with detox. These are just a few that I found most useful.

Colonics and Coffee Enemas

I found that colonics and coffee enemas are a powerful way to detox. According to the Gerson Cancer Therapy protocol, coffee helps the

---

*Since detoxification was a part of my Lyme treatment as well, some text in this section is drawn from the earlier book (chapter 5).

liver dump toxins that have accumulated in this organ of filtration (Gerson 2007).

Sodium Bicarbonate

It turns out that sodium bicarbonate (baking soda) acts as a natural antacid and antihistamine. It has been found to "restrain viral entry" and can help absorb waste in the blood (Mir et al. 2020). I had many an intuitive hit for baking soda, not just for hot baths, as recommended on page 93, but also for taking it internally. Try taking 1 teaspoon in water three times a day.

Detoxifying Heavy Metals

Heavy metals, which pollute both groundwater and air, can impair the proper functioning of our immune system. Lead, mercury, nickel, cadmium, and aluminum collect in the brain and other areas in the body and may be linked to Alzheimer's, Lyme, Parkinson's, and other diseases (Lavelle 2003). They can also collect in the prostate gland and lead to complications. I "saw" that heavy metals tend to accumulate in the glands, especially the prostate and pineal glands.

Detoxifying your body of heavy metals is critical for maximizing the efficiency of your immune system. Chelating agents will help, including cholestyramine and DMSO; many people have reported success with them (Sears 2013). Other heavy metal detoxifiers include zeolite and bentonite clays, charcoal, chlorella, and the grasses, particularly wheatgrass and barley grass. Homeopathy can also work wonders for heavy metal detox.

Find out what feels best for your body, and also find a good doctor with a heavy metal detox protocol that works for you.

Herbs and Other Plants for Detoxification

Plant-based remedies that are effective for all-around detoxification include apple pectin, cacao (raw), cardamom, carob, cilantro, cinnamon, mung beans, oatmeal, *Mucuna pruriens* (velvet bean) powder, resveratrol (from red grapes), and turkey tail and reishi mushrooms. These all help reverse bioaccumulation by helping pull heavy metals and other toxins out of the body. In addition, you can support your liver with milk thistle and dandelion (Mulrow et al. 2000). I make a powder blend of the above herbs, which I combine with dandelion root to support the liver. Again, because of histamine reactions you will have to be careful with certain herbs. Also check out the raw healing soup recipe in appendix 4 for a good detoxifier.

> I "saw" aluminum and other metals in my brain in several intuitive meditations, followed by most of the above mentioned detoxifiers as medicines to help remove metals from the brain.

Sweating

Any kind of sweating can help detox the body. Try saunas, infrared saunas, hot springs, hot baths, and sweat lodges. After that heat, massage yourself from the back and sides of the neck toward the shoulders, as described earlier in this chapter. Cross your arms across your chest, laying your fingers on your clavicles, and gently lift your arms up and down (Vairo et al. 2009). Always drink plenty of water after sweating, as it helps the body cleanse itself.

Fasting

Fasting has been found to increase autophagy (the ability of the body to break down dead cells and waste) and boost the immune system (Hannan 2020). Many who suffer from long-haul Covid have found success with fasting. Try a three-day or longer fast, ingesting only hot water, lemon juice, and stevia, or try intermittent fasting. You might also try other protocols, like a three-day melon fast or a coconut water and wheatgrass fast. But be careful if you already have low glucose levels.

I found fasting for three to five days to be tremendously helpful; my symptoms would often subside after a couple days of no food. It was a good reminder of how much the gut and histamine intolerance are involved with long Covid symptoms.

Clay, Mud, and Mineral Packs

Clays, zeolites, salt, and mud are great tools for detoxing the body. Many companies make products that do just this. You pack mud, for example, onto various parts of your body, including the feet and head, to draw out toxins through the skin (Moosavi 2017). You can also take certain clays and zeolites internally; just make sure you follow a qualified practitioner's protocol.

Liver and Gallbladder Flushes

The liver and gallbladder are some of the most crucial organs for healing toxicity. The liver is like the fuel oil tank, and the gallbladder is the regulator of that fuel, which is bile. Gallstones and backed-up bile can contribute to an overall breakdown of health in your body. The simplest gallbladder and liver flush I have found is the Hulda Clark liver and gallbladder flush, which consists of olive oil, grapefruit juice, apple juice, psyllium powder, and Epsom salts (Clark 1995). Specific instructions can be found online. I suggest doing a series of flushes for best results, as sometimes it can take a few times to get things moving. I did quite a few when I was sick and experienced nothing but benefits (although the olive oil can be nauseating).

Detox Baths

Taking hot baths with baking soda, clays, and Epsom salts can help the body detox. Try a hot bath with 1 to 2 cups of baking soda, 1 to 2 cups of Epsom salts, 1 cup of bentonite clay, and 1 cup of borax. Soak for 20 minutes. There are many other detox herbal bath blends you can try with herbs such as mustard and ginger. Also try including detox foot soaks in your routine.

VACCINE DETOXIFICATION

You'll find a lot of information and hearsay on the safety and efficacy of the vaccines. Some of the ingredients in the vaccine may indeed be toxic and some may be harmless. Without going down a rabbit hole,

I can only report what I experienced with the Pfizer-BioNTech and Johnson & Johnson vaccines.

I took the Pfizer-BioNTech vaccine about six months post-Covid to see if it would help with my long-hauler symptoms. After taking the vaccine I woke up in the night with horrible sensations and taste in my mouth. I remember thinking that the adjuvant or carrier intuitively "felt" like fermented pig's brain or something similarly nasty, or a very toxic manufactured chemical. Some say it's graphene oxide, a toxic chemical used as an adjuvant in some vaccines (Ou et al. 2016), but for the Covid vaccines, despite claims, there is no scientific evidence yet for this. (Although I did see an independent lab analysis claiming there was graphene oxide in Covid vaccines.) Whatever it was, I remember feeling quite disgusted and immediately had "hits" to detox it. In the end, this first vaccine shot did nothing for me. Six months later I took the Johnson & Johnson vaccine after a strong intuitive "hit" about it, and although it felt cleaner, I had the clear image of a white serum that was capable of tearing things, like it had shards of glass in it. In any case, the J&J vaccine did help reduce my symptoms, taking the edge off by about 25 percent, I'd say. Hey, I'll take it. My intuitive hits for detoxing the vaccine included charcoal, chlorella, chlorophyll, cilantro, coffee enemas, dandelion, foot baths, homeopathic Thuja, wheatgrass, and zeolites.

DETERGENTS, SOAPS, AND SAPONINS FOR DETOXIFYING SPIKE PROTEINS

As discussed previously, by far the biggest "hit" I had for getting at the spike proteins was soap and detergents: bars of soap, Windex, Ajax, bubbles, and even plants like agave that contain high levels of saponins (natural soaps). Again and again during my meditations I would see these (internally) toxic products. The question became: What is it in soaps and detergents that my body is needing? And what can I actually take that won't kill me? I started researching common ingredients in all of the detergents and soaps that I was seeing. Here's what I came up with.

Turns out bar soap is typically made from lye and animal fat. Lye, or sodium hydroxide, is used to break down proteins or amino acids. Guess who is a nasty little protein we want to break down? The spike protein. But how can we get soap into the body? After all, **lye is very toxic.** However, there are foods that are cooked with lye, and you can buy lye water (sodium hydroxide and water) online. It's often used in Asian foods like ramen and century eggs, but usually it's cooked off. I ordered some lye water and experimented with taking just a few drops a day with fat. I *don't* recommend this—and lye *must* be diluted before being consumed— but hey, when you're sick, you'll try anything.

Another approach could be MMS, "Miracle" or "Master" Mineral Solutions. The solution is made by combining sodium chlorite and hydrochloric acid or citric acid to get chlorine dioxide. Chlorine dioxide is a detergent and has been found to have antibiotic effect (Kim, Park, and Rhee 2014) as well as to be effective against Covid-19 (Hatanaka et al. 2021). According to my intuition, it breaks down the spike proteins. There are entire long Covid groups devoted to the use of chlorine dioxide and its benefits. **The FDA has recently come out with dire warnings against use of this product,** however, I believe it has benefits—but it must be used in very small amounts (no more than drops) and with utmost caution. See chapter 9 for more information.

Salt (sodium chloride) and baking soda (sodium bicaronate) also have natural detergent properties, and I had many intuitive "hits" for them. Try 1 teaspoon of either compound in water three times a day.

The other product with a detergent-like effect that I kept "seeing" is Coca-Cola, likely because of the phosphoric and citric acids. Think of coke like drain cleaner. **Phosphoric acid is toxic in large amounts. Please be very careful with any kind of chemical; the wrong combination can be disasterous or even lethal.** Other acids may have a spike-dissolving effect as well (see chapter 9).

What about plants that are naturally high in saponins? As

mentioned before, I had many intuitive hits for agave. It turns out that agaves have steroidal saponins with anti-neuroinflammatory properties, glucose-lowering properties, and immunomodulating properties (Herrera-Ruiz et al. 2021; Simmons-Boyce and Tinto 2007; Misra, Varma, and Kumar 2018), and I believe they can help break down and scrub out the spike protein trash. In addition, steroidal saponins exhibit cytotoxic effect on cancer cells through induction of apoptosis and help control protein expression linked to cancer progression and metastasis (Escobar-Sánchez, Sánchez-Sánchez, and Sandoval-Ramírez 2015). One particular steroidal saponin isolated from agave, called hecogenin, has been shown to be a potent immunomodulator, antifungal, and anti-inflammatory and effective at reducing the cytokine storm (Ingawale, Mandlik, and Patel 2019).

Other plants that have high levels of saponins include asparagus, horse chestnut, licorice, soapbark, and soapwort, among others. I have seen horse chestnut used in other long-haul protocols. Needless to say, I'm a big fan of saponins for long-haul Covid; we will discuss them more in chapter 9.

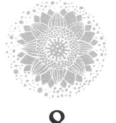

8

✦ ✦ ✦

Diet and Foods for Long Covid

Histamine Intolerance, Gut Health, Ketosis, and Other Considerations

ABOUT A MONTH AFTER MY INITIAL INFECTION WITH COVID, I began to get headaches and a kind of burning sensation in the frontal lobe area of my brain. It reminded me of a hay fever kind of headache, or histamine allergy feeling, except it never went away. Then I noticed that certain foods I was eating worsened my symptoms. I remember eating a can of sardines, and an hour later, whammo! Excruciating headache pain for hours. Turns out I and most long-haulers are dealing with mast cell activation syndrome (MCAS) and may develop a dietary histamine intolerance.

Diet becomes very important for long-haulers, though everyone reacts differently to the same foods. I discovered that a bland ketogenic diet coupled with a low-histamine diet, with a couple of exceptions, worked best for my body.

MAST CELL ACTIVATION SYNDROME (MCAS)

MCAS is an immunological condition in which mast cells, a type of white blood cell, excessively release chemical mediators, resulting in a range of chronic symptoms. This is a normal reaction in allergies, but in the case of long-haul Covid it becomes chronic. Primary symptoms include cardiovascular, dermatological, gastrointestinal, neurological, and respiratory problems as well as excessive histamine release. MCAS sets up the massive inflammatory response seen in long-haul Covid patients (Weinstock et al. 2021). Researchers are now finding that MCAS is more often than not triggered by mold overgrowth (Kritas et al. 2018).

> *For me it felt like my brain was always on fire; another sufferer of long Covid described it as "a sunburn on the brain."*

HISTAMINE OVERLOAD

When the immune system encounters a potential allergen, such as pollen, mold, or certain foods, mast cells release histamines into the bloodstream. Histamines boost blood flow in the area of your body the allergen has affected, which facilitates the flow of other chemicals from your immune system to the site for defense and repair. This causes inflammation, but it is all a normal process, and the histamines die down after the repair work is done. In long-haul Covid and other chronic illnesses, mast cells get stuck in a continuous loop of activation and keep releasing histamines. Perhaps, in the case of long Covid, the spike proteins lingering in your own white blood cells are the offending allergen as put forth by Dr. Bruce Patterson and team (Patterson et al. 2022a). In this case, you would essentially become allergic to your own blood. This is essentially mast cell activation syndrome.

With long Covid, perhaps because of the chronic histamine overload, we can develop sensitivities to foods high in histamine. Imagine that you have a histamine bucket. When you eat, any histamine in your food gets dumped in the bucket. If your bucket is already mostly full due to the fallout from long Covid, it will quickly overflow, leading to histamine reactivity. For these reasons, it's important to focus your diet on foods low in histamine, foods that liberate histamine, and foods that help lower histamine levels.

GUT HEALTH

Before we can explore the best diet for long-haulers, it is important to get the gut in tip-top shape. Rebuilding the lining of the gut is especially important, as described in chapter 6, not only for digestive health but also for immune health. I found the supplements and practices below to be helpful; see chapter 9, too, for a more complete list of antihistamines.

- **Diamine oxidase (DAO).** Take it as a supplement before eating to slow the histamine response. This enzyme helps break down histamine-rich foods and may reduce symptoms of histamine intolerance (Schnedl et al. 2019).
- **Supplements to rebuild the gut lining.** Try homeostatic soil organisms (HSO), fulvic acid, licorice, aloe vera, and L-glutamine.
- **Panax ginseng.** This Asian ginseng has been found to block histamines well (Jang et al. 2015). Try taking it before eating.
- **Probiotics.** Probiotics (and prebiotics) support gut health. Be sure to get a good low-histamine version. Some probiotics, such as those from ferments like kimchi and sauerkraut as well as dairy, may activate histamine. Specific probiotic formulations can now be catered to the individual based on a microbiome analysis. *Bacillus subtilis* has been found to have a direct effect on Covid-19 (Alam et al. 2021).
- **Enzymes.** Pancreatic enzymes, protease, amylase, lumbrokinase, serrapeptase, and other digestive ezymes are not only able to break down proteins (perhaps lingering spike proteins), they also break down carbohydrates and lipids, aiding the gut in proper digestion. However, interestingly, the Covid virus may actually use proteolytic enzymes to help spread itself around by cleaving the spike into two pieces (S1 and S2) (Gioia et al. 2020).

- **Breathwork.** Practice nauli, or abdominal churning, to stimulate the "fire" in the belly and your immune system. You can also try pranayama or the Breath of Fire exercise.
- **Emotional processing.** Work with any underlying emotional issues stuck in the gut, as discussed in chapter 4.
- **Foods to build inner fire.** Stoke your inner fire and support brain health by eating foods high in fats and grasses like wheatgrass. Avoid gluten, grains, and other immune-dampening foods. Eat a low-histamine modified ketogenic diet.
- **Sugar-free gum.** Chew sugar-free chewing gum to activate the release of amylase and other enzymes needed for the proper breakdown of food. Gum chewing also decreases anxiety levels and can help with mood (Sasaki-Otomaru et al. 2011).

THE LONG-HAUL DIET: KETOGENIC AND LOW-HISTAMINE

Ketogenic/Low-Carbohydrate Diet

The ketogenic diet, which is quite popular these days, basically cuts out carbs and sugars. The idea is to bring your body into ketosis, a state in which your body burns fat for fuel instead of carbohydrates. This form of low-carb diet helps reduce mast cells and histamine in the body (Nakamura et al. 2014). You can find much information and guidance on ketogenic diets online and in other books, so we won't get into the details here.

> Many times the word keto popped into my head, so I went with it and found the ketogenic diet helpful in reducing my symptoms. However, it becomes a bit tricky when you're also trying to eat a low-histamine diet, and I found that I had to combine and modify the two diets. My intuitive dietary list ended up looking like a combination of ketogenic and low-histamine foods, and overall leaning toward bland. This is a good place to start. I was able to reintroduce other foods as I got better.

Low-Histamine Diet

Histamine intolerances arise from an overaccumulation of histamine in the body. A low-histamine diet reduces the risk for reactivity. You will need to see what foods specifically affect you, but below are some general guidelines.

Foods to Avoid

- Junk food and processed foods (generally, the more processed a food, the more inflammatory it is)
- Aged cheeses
- Artificial preservatives (e.g., BHA, BHT, benzoates, sulfites)
- Artificial dyes (e.g., tartrazine/FD&C Yellow #5, which is also found in some medications and supplements)
- Artificial flavors (e.g., MSG and other glutamates)
- Foods with any trace of mold or spoilage
- Cured or aged meats (salami, sausage, hot dogs)
- Pickled foods and condiments
- Preserved foods, specifically anything canned or aged
- Smoked foods (e.g., smoked salmon)
- Sugary foods and drinks (sugar feeds unwelcome yeast and bacteria that can cause gut damage)
- Refined carbohyrates (e.g., white flour)
- Energy drinks
- Fermented foods and drinks (e.g., sauerkraut, kimchi, kombucha, soy sauce, yogurt)
- Gluten (e.g., wheat and rye)
- Nightshades (e.g., eggplant, spinach, tomatoes)
- Yeast, yeast extracts (e.g., Marmite and Vegemite), and yeast products (e.g., breads and pastries)
- Dried fruits (e.g., raisins, prunes, dates)
- Overripe foods (e.g., squishy or brown avocados)
- Some spices (cayenne, cinnamon, cloves, etc.; you can find complete lists of high-histamine spices online)

Many lists of foods for people with histamine intolerance to avoid also include the following foods, though reactivity to them is individual: dairy, eggs, citrus (oranges, mandarins), papaya, pineapples, strawberries, raspberries, bananas, pumpkin, soy, potatoes, lentils, beans (pulses), chocolate, cocoa, and some nuts.

Foods to Enjoy

These foods can all help you avoid or calm a histamine reaction. This is a generalized list, of course; you'll have to determine for yourself whether you are sensitive to any of the foods listed here.

- Fresh, organic, local (if possible) unprocessed foods
- Whole, fresh veggies and fruits (except bananas and citrus), especially cabbage, broccoli, cauliflower, artichoke, and all the greens
- Berries (e.g., blueberries and blackberries)
- Fresh foods and meats, or foods that are frozen fresh immediately after being harvested or prepared
- Foods rich in vitamin C (e.g., berries, apples, broccoli, onions, dandelion greens)
- Foods rich in vitamin B_2 (e.g., mushrooms, asparagus, eggs, almonds)
- Foods rich in vitamin B_6 (e.g., cabbage, cauliflower, sweet potato, liver, salmon)
- Foods rich in magnesium (leafy greens, almonds, dark chocolate)
- Foods rich in copper (nuts, seeds, shiitake and crimini mushrooms)
- Foods rich in zinc (nuts, seeds, meats, shellfish)
- Foods rich in omega-3 fatty acids (e.g., wild-caught, cold-water, frozen-at-sea or very fresh fish such as salmon, mahi, and halibut, as well as freshly ground flaxseed and chia seeds)
- Quality oils (e.g., organic, expeller-pressed extra virgin olive oil, grapeseed oil, avocado oil, and coconut oil; note that even when avocados are not tolerated, the oil usually is)

There are plenty of other histamine-lowering foods, which often contain quercetin and other antioxidants, like onions and apples.

Also I found that raw (unpasteurized) dairy products worked well for me, and there are studies confirming the anti-inflammatory and immunomodulatory effects of raw dairy (Sozańska 2019; Cross and Gill 2000).

The above list is a good place to start, but as noted earlier, we will all react differently. You will have to find what works for you. So that you can really know how different foods affect you, I suggest doing a two-day fast to reset your system. Then introduce foods one by one, wait a few hours, and note whether you had symptoms. Slowly but surely, you will build a list of safe foods.

Blood Glucose

Glucose is the main sugar found in your blood, and it is controlled by insulin, a hormone created by the pancreas. The brain inflammation caused by Covid can interfere with hormone signaling and dysregulate the body's insulin response, leading to increased glucose levels in the body (Montefusco et al. 2021).

Once again, reducing inflammation becomes paramount; see chapter 5. There are medicines and foods that can help reduce blood sugar levels, such as metformin (by prescription), nopal cactus, special probiotics, and chromium picolinate among others (Ali et al. 2011), and we'll discuss them in chapter 9. Also important is a low-sugar diet; eating a ketogenic diet will help with this.

> My glucose levels were normal before Covid. Interestingly, once I developed long-haul Covid, I had a number of intuitive "hits" to eat some sugars. I would often have intuitive downloads for molasses, cantaloupe, and watermelon. One day my wife put her hand on my head and said, "Your brain needs sugar." Turns out the brain needs sugar.

The brain needs a tremendous amount of glucose to function and is the main consumer of glucose in the body. If this metabolic pathway is disrupted, brain diseases can occur. However, excess glucose in the brain can cause memory and cognitive deficiencies (Mergenthaler et al. 2013). With long Covid, we have an altered cerebral glucose metabolism (Hosp et al. 2021), so it may be that sugar is not being properly metabolized and builds up in the blood. I think that there is something going on with fat (high cholesterol) blocking sugars from entering cells, a metabolism issue.

> *I did some research on what I was intuiting and it turns out that molasses occasionally helped my headaches, cantaloupe and watermelon are low on the glycemic index, and cantaloupe can also help with the metabolism of glucose (Park 2021). I also often had images of nopales, or opuntia cactus, turns out opuntia is great for lowering blood sugar (Hwang, Kang, and Lim 2017). My needs might be very different from yours, but it's important to trust your body's wisdom on what foods you may need or not. I chose to listen to what my body was telling me, and I always checked in with an expert on what I was intuiting.*

Other Considerations

Long Covid may cause other kinds of food intolerances to develop, such as sensitivities to foods with high levels of salicylates or oxalatesm like turmeric, prunes, and cayenne. I found that eating more than one chicken egg would negatively affect me, for some reason, as would turmeric deriviatives and supplements such as curcumin; fresh turmeric with milk seemed fine, though. If you suspect a particular food is affecting you, listen to your body.

• •

Food Diary

Over the course of my experience with long Covid, I kept a food diary. I had to figure out my own best diet through trial and error. Some days would be so painful if I ate the wrong foods, and I would often have symptoms for days. Other times I could reach a tolerable baseline (about 70 percent of normal) if I ate the right things.

You should keep your own diary, too, not only for foods but also for supplements and medicines, tracking your reactions and your own intuitive "hits." The foods that are healing for your body will be different from those that are healing for mine.

Here's what came up for me as the most important foods for *my* body:

- Oils (hot oils were best): omega-3 fatty acids, fish oil (like EPA-rich oil from salmon); University of Illinois at Chicago 2019), medium-chain triglyceride (MCT) oil, coconut oil, hemp oil, evening primrose oil, olive oil, black currant oil, black cumin seed (*Nigella sativa*) oil, sea buckthorn oil, walnut oil, mustard oil, grapeseed oil, macadamia oil, sesame oil (Li et al. 2016)
- Other fats (hot and fresh were best; with care if LDL cholesterol levels are high): butter (ghee), buttermilk (sips), pork fat (organic), cacao butter, raw cream, raw milk/colostrum (try goat)
- Fresh bone broths (be careful as bone broth can be aged), collagen, chicken cartilage, chicken soup
- Fruits: pomegranates, blueberries, blackberries, watermelon, cantaloupe, green apples
- Nuts: raw pecans, walnuts, and Brazil nuts
- Veggies: onion, garlic, broccoli, cauliflower, all greens (except spinach), avocado, beets, carrots, peas, celery, artichoke, cabbage
- Oats (these aren't ketogenic but I kept having "hits" for them so I went with it)
- Beans: fresh white or kidney beans
- Condiments and spices: mayonnaise, mustard, coffee (try a quarter or half cup), ginger, cayenne, horseradish, black pepper, cumin, honey, spearmint and mint
- Meats (not smoked): fish, chicken, turkey, bison, beef, game
- Eggs: just one chicken egg at a time; duck eggs were good, too
- Alchohol: wine, mescal (I had strong "hits" that alchohol breaks the spike proteins; see chapter 9)

FASTING

As discussed in chapter 7, a number of studies indicate that fasting or intermittent fasting can be helpful for detoxifying the body, and they can also help reduce the severity of MCAS (Nakamura et al. 2014). Fasting can also be a good way to clear your body of potential allergens so that you can then reintroduce foods one by one and identify which are triggering a reaction.

PUTTING YOUR DIET TOGETHER

It can be daunting and incredibly frustrating to have to change your diet, sometimes dramatically, and especially when you're trying to find out what triggers very painful, days-long reactions. I remember being terrified to try something new, just praying I wouldn't react later. But you have to stay strong. You have to become a food warrior and find out what works best for you, using trial and error and your intuition.

It can be hard when the family is cooking up a delicious pot of spaghetti with all the fixings. I can't tell you how many times I broke down and then later suffered, to the point of tears.

You can do it. You have to do it. Getting food intolerance and histamine response under control is a huge part of helping calm the storm. Get that diary going, let your family know, and stay disciplined and focused. And it's okay if you mess up; we all do, but try again until you succeed.

Affirmations

I easily and gently break down this food with no problems.

I absorb this nourishment with love.

I bless this food that is just right for my body.

I listen to my gut and am guided to what to eat.

I am focused and disciplined and eat foods that are healing for my body.

9

✦ ✦ ✦

The Medicines and Methods

An Integrative Approach

A GREAT DEAL OF RESEARCH IS UNDER WAY in the search for treatments for long-haul Covid. As we know, there are no miracle cures or (at the time of this writing) even broad consensus on the best approach. However, many people have healed from this chronic disease, sometimes pioneering new treatments, both mainstream and underground. And we can learn from their experience.

In this chapter I take a comprehensive approach, presenting everything from Western pharmacuticals to herbs to homeopathics to dissociative drugs to compounds and supplements. I found the integrative approach worked best for me, utilizing all the tools in the toolbox. In appendix 1 you can find my own narrowed down protocol.

As I worked through long Covid, I kept a diary where I recorded my intuitive "hits," research, and responses to treatment. I worked not just with my intuition but also with medical professionals. At the same time, I gathered information from other success stories and Covid forums, as well as keeping up with the evolving scientific investigations into long-haul Covid.

After some time, a treatment protocol emerged, mostly based on my intuition but also from the help of excellent doctors and healers. I present the medicines in this chapter. As I am not a doctor, I avoid listing dosages, leaving that up to you and your doctor. I *do* point out those substances that can be toxic. Keep in mind that although the information here is quite extensive, it is by no means comprehensive, and much more remains to be discovered.

For the sake of simplicity, I have divided the remedies and methods into categories based on function—that is, immune support and modulation, spike protein breakdown, anti-inflammatories, and so on. For each category, I list the possible remedies, everything from prescription pharmaceuticals to homeopathics to herbs and more. In general, I have listed the medicines and remedies in order of their importance to me personally. Where possible, I've annotated the remedies with studies, research, and explanations. Some of the recommendations are scientifically unsupported (yet!) or lack sufficient evidence of efficacy.

Remember that one person's medicine is another person's poison. This protocol is meant only as a guideline and to provide potential options. There are many different roads to healing. I encourage you to look through these lists and try the remedies that jump out at you. Use what works for you. Long Covid is a multifaceted illness, and you will need a comprehensive approach; I recommend employing one or two remedies from each category. For those who find all of these options overwhelming, skip to the section "Develop Your Treatment Protocol" for a simpler approach. You will need to stay focused and disciplined with your protocol. And remember to go back and hone your own intuitive skills.

A hodgepodge of remedies may clash with each other or cancel each other out. I encourage you to work with a medical professional who specializes in long-haul Covid to help design your protocol. This comprehensive overview may prove helpful not only to patients but to doctors as well. I also encourage you to *rotate* medicines from categories, look for *synergies,* and look for the magic or *alchemy.*

IMMUNE SUPPORT AND MODULATION

Here we look at medicines and techniques that smarten, calm, modulate, and reset the immune system. By "reset" I'm referring to treatments that can help the limbic system out of the trauma loop and calm the hyperactive immune response to the spike proteins.

1. Pharmaceuticals

- Ivermectin, which has immunomodulatory properties (Bryant et al. 2021) and can block spike proteins from entering the ACE-2 receptors, thereby decreasing further damage (Lehrer and Rheinstein 2020). Despite the controversy about it, there are literally hundreds of scientific articles on the efficacy of ivermectin for Covid. I know personally many people who say they were fully "cured' of long Covid with ivermectin as their main medicine. I found ivermectin helpful, as have others, and as many doctors who use it will tell you. However, for me it was not a magic bullet. It works best in conjunction with other medications like doxycycline or low-dose naltrexone (Mahmud et al. 2021).
- Low-dose naltrexone (Sims 2022). Calms the immune system, making it a very important medicine for long Covid and other diseases driven by an overactive immune system. This is one of the main medicines in the FLCCC protocol and has helped many with long-haul Covid. Personally, it didn't seem to help me much.
- Specialized pro-resolving mediators (SPMs) are regulators of inflammation, which are also helpful for infection (Basil and Levy 2016).

There are many other drugs that have immune suppessing abilities, such as hydroxychloroquine, steroids (discussed below), NSAIDS, azathioprine, and more. In many ways long-haul Covid resembles the disease lupus, and quite a few drugs that work for lupus have some effect with long Covid (Ramachandran 2022). Please check with your doctor.

2. Herbs

- Medicinal mushrooms, such as reishi and its constituent beta-glucan (Alhazmi et al. 2021), chaga, agarikon, turkey tail, shiitake, *Agaricus blazei,* lion's mane, and *Cordyceps militaris* (Hetland et al. 2021) all have important immune-modulating capabilities

(Guggenheim et al. 2014). Many of the mushrooms may also have anti-inflammatory, antihistamine, and other benefits. My personal favorites—which I place near the top of my list for long Covid medicines—are rieshi, lion's mane, agarikon, and turkey tail. (See my "Immune-Boosting Mushroom Milk" in appendix 4.)

- Immune apoptogenic herbs, like ashwagandha (Vetvicka and Vetvickova 2011), carnivora or Venus fly trap (Rowen 2013), shilajit—also for humic and fluvic acid (Musthafa et al. 2016), and garlic (Schäfer and Kaschula 2014)

3. Other Compounds

- Colostrum, which also has immunomodulatory effects thanks to its immunoglobulin G (Arenas et al. 2021; Rathe et al. 2014). Also try transfer factors (from colostrum and egg yolk) or lactoferrin.
- Intravenous immunoglobulin (IVIg) therapy. This is basically getting injected with antibodies from another person who was able to heal from Covid (Nguyen et al. 2020). In other words, it helps smarten your immune system. There is some evidence of IVIg being helpful for long Covid when used in combination with other drugs like steroids (Kindgen-Milles et al. 2022).

4. Psychedelics, Animal Medicines, and Dissociative Medicines

Only embark with a qualified practitioner—see chapter 10 for a full discussion.

- Kambo, a powerful toxin from a South American frog used in various indigenous tribes. Kambo contains peptides, antimicrobial and anti-inflammatory compounds (Hesselink 2018). There are now qualified practitioners in the United States (*International New York Times* 2021). I did a few sessions and it was very helpful.
- Dissociative medicines, such as ketamine, which also helps with depression (Sims 2022; Niciu et al. 2014); the synthetic 5MEO (Hu et al. 2021); ibogaine (House, Thomas, and Bhargava 1995);

ayahuasca; San Pedro cactus; psychedelic mushrooms; LSD; and peyote (Szabo 2015). All of these can also be microdosed and can have a mood enhancing effect. Paul Stamets, mycologist and lecturer, has championed the "Stamets Stack," which is combining lion's mane mushrooms with niacin and a microdose of psilocybin. Check the legality, scarcity, and cultural heritage of these medicines in your state or country, and proceed with the utmost caution and the assistance of a doctor, shaman, or certified practitioner.

5. *Homeopathics*

- Homeopathic formulations of any of the psychedelic and dissociative medicines listed above
- Homeopathic reptile remedies, like Crotalus, for calming the limbic system

• •

Homeopathics for Long-Haul Covid

Homeopathy can be of great benefit for long Covid. Homeopathics are vibrational remedies, or very tiny amounts of a substance working in a way of "like cures like," like the phenomenon of phase cancellation in music. Homeopathics are especially useful when you want to work with poisons or toxins like rattlesnake venom, whose homeopathic version is called Crotalus.

Homeopaths work in two ways: "Classical" homeopaths look for one high-potency remedy that will heal, like an IM potency. "Modern" homeopaths use lower potency for more symptomatic complaints, like Rhus toxicodendron (poison oak) 30C for a rash or similar complaint. The homeopathics listed in this chapter are all 200C and under. I encourage you to work with a classical homeopath for a deeper dive. I've seen and experienced miracles with homeopathy.

Please see appendix 5 for a full list of remedies and their actions for long-haul Covid. If you are working with the remedies yourself, order from a reputable supplier, like Hahnemann Labs, Helios Homeopathy (in the UK), or Washington Homeopathic Products.

• •

SPIKE PROTEIN BREAKDOWN

The lingering spike protein theory may in fact be the smoking gun of long Covid, or at least a big piece of the puzzle. Recall that the spike protein is really a glycoprotein, or a chain of amino acids with a coating of sugar around it. I "saw" the spike protein, as mentioned previously, and also remedies for breaking it down, which I've listed here. Please note that at the time of this writing some of these remedies are experimental or anecdotal. Fortunately some of the intuitive information I initially received about the spike proteins has since been validated by scientific research.

1. Detergents

See the discussion in chapter 7. Some of the following products are extremely *caustic* and *toxic* and must be used with the utmost care. Despite the FDA warnings of taking detergents internally, all of the following have been found to kill the virus in external applications. If you do consume these products, always use just a few drops and diluted. Better yet, look for these as homeopathics. A number of people have been hurt by these detergents—mostly from taking large amounts—and I again urge the utmost caution.

- Chlorine dioxide has been found to inhibit spike proteins on ACE-2 receptors (Ogata and Miura 2021). When you combine sodium chlorite and hydrochloric acid or citric acid this forms chlorine dioxide. Some people consume sodium chlorite and allow the acids of the stomach (HCL) to create the reaction. Despite the controversy and warnings from the FDA on its toxicity. I found this to be quite effective and believe it made a big difference in my healing. Other groups and persons have also touted it as being very effective. Again, those who consume it should use only a few drops, diluted.
- Sodium hydroxide (lye) or lye water breaks down proteins (Høstmark, Sørensen, and Askevold 1977). Those who consume it should use no more than a few drops, diluted, and with fat.
- Sodium chloride (salt) is a natural detergent as well and has been

found to decrease viral load (Yang et al. 2020). I had many intuitive hits for salt for "washing" the brain and place it high on my list. Again use small amounts—no more than ½ teaspoon at a time—as it can be a purgative in large amounts. There are also effective salt supplements for redox signaling.

- Borax is actually a salt but has been used in detergent products. Some long-haul sufferers claim it can detox the spike proteins. I never tried it.
- Detox foot baths. Baking soda, Borax, and Clorox can all be used as detox foot baths and have been used to pull pesticides out of the body. Use very small amounts, or go swimming or hot tubbing in pools treated with chlorine.
- Calcium carbonate. One of the main ingredients of Ajax is actually calcium carbonate. Calcium carbonate can be taken internally safely and is found as a supplement. Try also the homeopathic remedy Calc. Carb.

2. Soaps and Saponins

Soaps break down proteins into amino acids, and they were the biggest intuitive "hit" I had along with detergents. As discussed in chapter 7, I would often have images of the agave plant with bars of soap. This leads us to plant-derived steroidal saponins, which are soaps, and my number one remedy for long haul Covid. They also help with inflammation as discussed previously. Plants with high levels of saponins include the following:

- Agave (Simmons-Boyce and Tinto 2007) and its constituent hecogenin
- Licorice
- Horse chestnut (Yokosuka et al. 2000; Puttaswamy et al. 2020)
- Aloe
- Sea buckthorn (Zhan et al. 2021)
- Soapbark (*Quillaja saponaria*); also used as an adjuvent in vaccines
- Soapwort (*Saponaria officinalis*)

3. Enzymes

Enzymes can break down proteins and they may also break down the spike proteins and help with blood clots.

- Nattokinase derived from earthworms
- Lumbrokinase (Farhadi et al. 2018)
- Protease
- Serrapeptase
- Glycoside hydrolase enzymes (alpha- and beta-galactosidase, etc.)
- Pancreatic enzymes
- Pepsin
- Trypsin
- Elastase
- Chymotrypsin (Gioia et al. 2020)

4. Herbs and Essential Oils

I had an intuitive "hit" that the terpenes in some essential oils can break down the spike proteins.

- Licorice, which has shown activity against spike proteins (Yu et al. 2021)
- Rosemary essential oil has lots of terpenes; nebulize it.
- Tea tree essential oil, which is also antiviral, also has lots of terpenes (Patne, Mahore, and Tokmurke 2020)

5. Homeopathics

Homeopathics are one of my favorite ways (and non-toxic) to get at the spike proteins.

> I had a very clear vision of broken glass in what looked like soy sauce. This to me says silica (glass) breaks down proteins into chains of amino acids (soy sauce). I also had many images of pencils (graphite) and rubber tires (petroleum or latex). The homeopathic remedies Silicea 30C, Graphites 6C, and Petroleum 6C became important allies.

- Silicea 30C
- Graphites 6C
- Petroleum 6C
- China 30C
- Thuja 30C
- Causticum
- Natrum causticum (sodium hydroxide)
- Carcinosinum

6. Other Options

- Aminoglycoside antibiotics, like paromomycin. One day I "heard" the word *aminoglycosides* and it turns out that paromomycin inhibits the spike protein (Tariq et al. 2020).
- Acids. Acids can break down proteins. Anecdotal evidence relates that shikimic acid can break down the spike proteins and acts as an anticoagulant (Xiao-yl et al. 2014; Bochkov et al. 2012). It's present in pine needles, fennel, star anise, sprouts and more; prepare these remedies as a tea, or just eat fennel seeds. Other acids such as uric acid, nicotinic acid, and hydrochloric acid can all break down proteins. Hyaluronic acid can also bind to proteins. Fulvic acid (Winkler and Ghosh 2018) and humic acid are also important for reducing inflammation and blood sugar levels.
- Alcohol also breaks down proteins (AAT Bioquest 2020), and I kept "seeing" alcohol for eliminating spike proteins. It may trigger a histamine reaction, though, so proceed slowly. Try two drinks a week to start. Mescal and wine worked best for me.
- Turpentine, or terpenes, which breaks down proteins (Wusteman, Wight, Elia 1990). Try just a drop in water.

In addition, scientists are working on finding specific peptides that can disable the spike protein (Chatterjee et al. 2020) (see page 121).

MONOCYTE RECEPTOR BLOCKERS / IMMUNE CHECKPOINT INHIBITORS

As described in chapter 1, Dr. Bruce Patterson and his team of researchers have discovered lingering spike proteins in a type of white blood cell called nonclassical monocytes up to fifteen months after the onset of infection (Patterson et al. 2022a). Their approach to treatment is to block these monocytes with the spike proteins in them from docking on receptors on blood vessel walls—the CCR5 and fractalkine receptors—where they cause an allergic response and corresponding inflammation. The main blockers or antagonists that Dr. Patterson uses for these receptors are the drugs Maraviroc (for CCR5 receptor) and statins such as Atorvistatin (for fractalkine receptor), which are both approved by the US Food and Drug Administration (FDA). These drugs are not yet an FDA-approved treatment for long-haul Covid, but they may be by the time you read this. Many other CCR5 antagonists have been found through the course of HIV research, as that virus uses the same receptor. I list these below.

Another angle is the use of immune checkpoint inhibitors. Immune checkpoints are proteins that can turn immune T cells off or on. With long-haul Covid the immune system becomes dysregulated when immune checkpoints turn on autoantibodies that attack the self. Drugs called PD-1 blockers can potentially restore the immune system by blocking these proteins (Loretelli et al. 2021).

1. ACE-2 Blockers

The Covid virus initially gains entry via the ACE-2 receptor sites, as previously discussed. The ACE-2 blockers listed below may work best in the initial phase of infection.

Pharmaceuticals

- Ivermectin (Choudhury et al. 2021).
- Hydroxychloroquine and chloroquine (N. Wang et al. 2020).

2. CCR5 Blockers

Pharmaceuticals

- Maraviroc, an immunomodulator that blocks the autoimmune response via CCR5 (Risner et al. 2020; Sayana and Khanlou 2009; Patterson et al. 2022c)
- Angiotensin II receptor blockers, like Benicar, which are useful against autoantibodies (Arthur et al. 2021)
- KAND567 (Abdelmoaty et al. 2019)
- Anibamine, a pharmaceutical derived from rosewood *(Aniba citrifolia)*; (Zhang et al. 2010)

Chemical Compounds

- Peptide T (Redwine et al. 1999). Research on other peptides is ongoing (Wang et al. 2011).
- Small molecule compounds, like Tak-779, a CCR5 antagonist. Research for new CCR5 antagonists among the small chemical compounds is ongoing (Baba et al. 1999).
- Triterpene saponins (Barroso-González et al. 2009; Moses, Papadopoulou, and Osbourn 2014)

Herbs

- Curcumin, which is helpful for inflammation as well (Giri, Rajagopal, and Kalra 2004)
- Shikonin, known as zicao in traditional Chinese medicine, derived from purple gromwell *(Lithospermum erythrorhizon)*; (Chen et al. 2003)
- *Sanguisorba officinalis,* whose root, called di yu in traditional Chinese medicine, is used in the treatment of HIV (Liang et al. 2013)

3. Fractalkine Blockers

Pharmaceuticals

- Statins: Atorvastatin and many other pharmaceutical statins (Nabatov et al. 2007).

- Aspirin (Noels and Weber 2010)
- Lovastatin (derived from red yeast rice and oyster mushrooms)

Chemical Compounds
- Niacin

Herbs
- Garlic (Sorrentino 2012)
- Nopal cactus
- Psyllium

ANTI-INFLAMMATORIES

Anti-inflammatories have some overlapping effects with antihistamines (see page 122) and immune modulators but act in a different manner. There are many more anti-inflammatories waiting to be discovered. These are just a few that worked for me.

1. Pharmaceuticals
- NSAIDs. Aspirin seemed to work best for my body. I had many intuitive hits for aspirin and place it high on my list.
- Fluvoxamine. An SSRI normally used for mood (see page 135), it has an immunomodulating effect that helps calm inflammation as well (Sukhatme et al. 2021). Be very careful when weaning off of it, you must do it slowly over weeks. Consult with your doctor.
- Montelukast, which is also used for asthma (try using it in combination with Xyzal); (Barré, Sabatier, and Annweiler 2020; May and Gallivan 2022). I have friends who say this helped and others who said it made things worse.

2. Steroids
Use with caution and by prescription only. Try a tapering dose or, as the Front Line COVID-19 Critical Care Alliance (FLCCC) recommends, a continuous low dose for a week or longer (Lin et al. 2021; Front Line COVID-19 Critical Care Alliance 2022).

- Prednisone. I had "hits" for this and took a low-dose course for ten days. It was helpful.
- Dexamethasone. Another useful steroid.

3. Oils

I had many intuitive hits for the following oils as hot oils, meaning that we can heat them up for better absorption. They are powerful anti-inflammatories and are at the top of my list for help with inflammation. Here are the ones I found most effective:

- Black currant seed oil
- Black seed *(Nigella sativa)* oil (Ahmad et al. 2013)
- Sea buckthorn oil (Zielińska and Nowak 2017)
- Olive oil
- Avocado oil
- Fish oil (omega-3)
- Grapeseed oil

4. Herbs/Supplements
- Andrographis has a strong anti-inflammatory effect (Zou et al. 2016)
- Resveratrol (Ramdani and Bachari 2020) (see page 126)
- CBD oil. Cannabis without THC is also a potent anti-inflammatory (Poudel et al. 2021). I had many intuitive hits for this and place it high on my list. And no, you don't get high with CBD.
- Curcumin (Thimmulappa et al. 2021) (try fresh turmeric)
- Bromelain (Sagar et al. 2020) (see page 123)
- Aloe vera also helps with the gut lining
- Opuntia. Also a great plant for lowering glucose levels. I had a lot of "hits" for this.
- Sage (*Salvia* genus)
- Dragon's blood
- Garlic, which is also an important immunomodulator (Schäfer and Kaschula 2014)

- Chuchuasi (*Maytenus laevis*). In addition to having strong anti-inflammatory effects it has been found to have anti-tumor effects (Gonzales et al. 1982). I found it an effective anti-inflammatory for Covid.
- Yarrow (*Achillea millefolium*). In addition to being an anti-inflammatory herb, yarrow is a great plant for stopping bleeding and healing wounds. It has been shown to aid brain disorders such as multiple sclerosis and neurogenerative disorders (Ayoobi et al. 2017).
- Boswellia. A potent anti-inflammatory and antihistamine (Siddiqui 2011).
- Various Chinese formulas. Consult with a specialist.

. . . .

Chinese Medicine

Traditional Chinese medicine (TCM) has a long history of use in China and other Asian countries, such as Japan and Korea. TCM is part of mainstream medicine in these countries and is frequently used by Americans who have roots in these traditions of healing. Herbal therapy and acupuncture are the main components of TCM. TCM herbal medicines are considered dietary supplements in the United States. There are hundreds of formulas that have been carefully constructed over thousands of years. If you feel called to go this route, there are many TCM practioners in North America and elsewhere.

. . . .

5. Saponins and Steroidal Saponins

The anti-inflammatory, antidiabetic, immunomodulating, and detoxification effects of saponins (natural soaps) have been extensively reported (Ejelonu et al. 2017; Herrera-Ruiz et al. 2021; Misra, Varma, and Kumar 2018).

- Soapworts (*Saponaria* species), which are normally used for bronchitis and inflammation, are high in saponins.

- Soapbark (*Quillaja saponaria*), an antiviral that is also high in saponins, is used as an adjuvant in vaccines (NovaVax) (Roner et al. 2007)
- Agave (Simmons-Boyce and Tinto 2007) and its constituent hecogenin
- Aloe. Beneficial for the gut. The skin of the plant has the highest saponins.
- Licorice is also beneficial for the gut.
- Horse chestnut (*Aesculus hippocastanum*) is normally used to reduce fevers and alleviate coughs. It can also be used for blood clots and is high in saponins (Dudek Makuch and Studzińska-Sroka 2015).
- Yucca is an anti-inflammatory high in saponins (Monterrosas-Brisson et al. 2013; Sánchez, Heredia, and García 2005)

6. Peptides

These are potent anti-inflammatory, immunomodulating, and anti-microbial compounds. They are typically injected with an insulin needle. Some peptides, such as NAD, can be quite expensive. Be on the lookout for new peptides for long-haul Covid, as I believe they are the medicine of the future.

- Nicotinamide adenine dinucleotide (NAD)
- Vasoactive intestinal polypeptide (VIP)
- LL-37
- Humanin (Beshay et al. 2021)
- Cerebrolysin
- BPC-157 (Chang et al. 2011)
- Thymosin alpha-1 (TA1)
- LL-3 (Mahendran et al. 2020)
- Hecogenin, from the agave plant (Ingawale and Patel 2016)
- Bee and wasp venom peptides, which are also bioregulators (Jafar et al. 2016)
- Phosphatidylcholine

7. Gases

- Hyperbaric oxygen has been found to be very effective for long-haul Covid (Kjellberg, De Maio, and Lindholm 2020).
- Ozone (see page 129)
- Hydrogen (in hydrogen peroxide; see page 128), also as a supplement where one adds a tablet to water. Hydrogen gas has also been suggested as an effective treatment for Covid according to some studies (Y. Li et al. 2021).

8. Other Options

- Stem cells, which regulate inflammation
- Myo-inositol (vitamin B_8), a sugar that can help with glucose levels, downregulate inflammation in Covid, and have a positive effect on mood (Bizzarri et al. 2020)
- Microdose psychedelics, such as LSD, peyote, San Pedro cactus, psilocybin, or synthetic psilocybin. This can be helpful for reducing inflammation, disrupting the limbic system trauma loop, relieving headaches, and stimulating the growth of new neurons (Andersson, Persson, and Kjellgren 2017; Flanagan and Nichols 2018). Check the legality in your state or country, of course.

ANTIHISTAMINES

These all help with mast cell activation and histamine overload. Combinations of H1 and H2 antihistamines have been shown to be most effective (Bhattacharyya 2020). Or perhaps you might consider upping the dosage on standard antihistamines—*work with a qualified doctor and always use caution.* Your diet will be key here; use the antihistamines as symptoms present.

1. Pharmaceuticals

- H1 Antihistamines: cetirizine (Zyrtec, Xyzal); loratadine (Claritin, Benadryl, etc.). Try combinations with H2 antihistamines and see what works best for you. Zyrtec worked best for me.

- H2 antihistamines: famotidine (Pepcid, Zantac, etc.). I had a hit for Pepcid early on and found it invaluable to help with my brain-burning symptoms.
- Ketotifen. Really a mast cell stabilizer, ketotifen works like an antihistamine and helped me quite a bit. It requires a prescription.
- Cromolyn sodium. Another mast cell stabilizer that can be very helpful for long Covid histamine (Yousefi et al. 2021; Bennett 2020; Malone et al. 2020). I know people who say this worked really well for them. It can be very expensive.

2. *Natural Antihistamines*

- Quercetin (Saeedi-Boroujeni and Mahmoudian-Sani 2021; Mlcek et al. 2016). I had many intuitive "hits" for quercetin. It is invaluable for long-haul Covid.
- Skullcap. One of my favorite herbal antihistamines. Try it with Pepcid.
- Turmeric or curcumin (Kurup and Barrios 2008). Curiously, curcumin (turmeric extract) would bring on histamine symptoms in my body. Then I tried fresh turmeric with milk in a blender—like the traditional golden milk of India—and that did the trick.
- Nettles have a natural antihistamine effect (Kumaki et al. 2011)
- Bromelain, from pineapple, can be a powerful antihistamine and anti-inflammatory (Sagar et al. 2020). Be careful; pineapple can also cause a histamine reaction in some people.
- Korean perilla, found in the mint family, can help with histamine and asthma (*Perilla frutescens*) (Shin et al. 2000).
- Panax ginseng has been found to inhibit the histamine response (Wang et al. 2017). Try it before eating food.
- Ephedra (ma huang), or synthetic ephedrine, reduces swelling and acts as an antihistamine (Laccourreye et al. 2015). The herb is now illegal, and the synthetic requires a prescription. I found it helpful with long Covid.
- Lobelia. Lobelia is used for asthma and the lungs. In addition to being an antihistamine and anti-inflammatory, it has a regulating

effect on the immune system (Brown et al. 2016). I had many "hits" for lobelia; it has a similar qualtity to tobacco.

- Many essential oils, such as lavender, chamomile, tea tree, and peppermint act as antihistamines, including my favorite: rosemary (Choi et al. 2016). I had a strong intuitive hit for it.

3. Other Compounds

- Baking soda, a.k.a. sodium bicarbonate, acts as a natural antihistamine and detoxifier (Joly et al. 2000). I had many hits for baking soda and place it high on my list. I mixed a ½ teaspoon in water and drank it.
- Vitamin C has a long history of use as an effective antihistamine. Try mixing it with ¼ teaspoon of baking soda in water. I did this often and found it very helpful. I would also add ¼ teaspoon of salt to this mixture and drank it twice a day.
- Bee and wasp venom peptides can have an antihistamine effect (Jafar et al. 2016)

4. Homeopathics

- Histaminum
- Apis
- Rhus toxicodendron

ANTIMICROBIALS/ANTIVIRALS

As discussed in chapter 1, long Covid is likely no longer an infection of a replicating virus (although that is still possible for a few months following infection) but a disease of inflammation and immune dysregulation, so many antimicrobials will not be of much benefit. However, as noted in our earlier discussions, other infections like Lyme and those caused by the herpesvirus family (Epstein-Barr, varicella, etc.) as well as parasites and mold, can flare up, and some antimicrobials may help for them. There are, of course, many more antimicrobial and antivirals not listed here. These are the ones that I believe to be the most beneficial, based either on my research or personal experience—or both! Keep in mind that many Western pharmaceuticals have been repurposed for long-haul Covid and may have been originally used for something entirely different.

Use this section when you think you have a lingering infection of some sort. Please work with a doctor or practitioner who knows his or her stuff to determine dosages. I recommend rotation of these remedies, and I don't recommend using more than two antimicrobials at a time.

1. Western Pharmaceuticals

- Ivermectin is an antiparasitic, anti-inflammatory compound (see also page 109).*
- Hydroxychloroquine. There is some evidence pointing to this antiparasitic and immunosuppressive drug helping with long Covid, also when combined with the antibiotic azithromycin, but solid science is lacking (Ip et al. 2021). However, the Front Line COVID-19 Critical Care Alliance has found that hydroxychloroquine has a strong effect for acute Covid and the newer omicron variants and recommend it on their website as a second line therapy for long Covid.
- Suramin. This is another anti-parasitic drug for nematode worms (used to treat the tropical disease river blindness) that has been found to inhibit Covid in vitro (Eberle et al. 2021). I took it for a couple of months with perhaps some effect.
- Nitazoxanide (Alinia). This may help with spike proteins in long-haul Covid; it also gets at the cysts in Lyme disease (Blum et al. 2021). Dr. Dietrich Klinghardt, a leading Lyme and long Covid doctor, places it high on his list for "persister cells;" according to his website it may get at the spike proteins.

---

*Interestingly, the traditional use of ivermectin has a strong effect on killing nematode worms (Strongyloides). According to the work and research of Dr. Alan MacDonald these worms happen to harbor viruses and bacteria, including Lyme disease. He found these worms not only in Lyme sufferers but also in patients with multiple sclerosis (MacDonald 2016). I wrote about this in my book on Lyme disease.

- Colchicine. Normally used for gout and rheumatic inflammation, this drug has been found to have an anti-inflammatory effect for Covid (Reyes et al. 2021).
- Paromomycin. An aminoglycoside antibiotic used for parasites (amoebas), paromomycin was found to inhibit spike proteins (Tariq et al. 2020).
- Other useful antibiotics—amoxicillin, azithromycin, doxycycline. There is some scientific evidence that these antibiotics can help with long-haul Covid in combination with other drugs like hydroxychloroquine (FLCCC 2022).

> *I think antibiotics are helpful for long-haul Covid when other bacteria have flared—such as Lyme disease or gut dysbiosis. I had a "hit" about amoxicillin helping to knock back some bad gut bugs. I took a two-week course and found it helpful.*

- Mebendazole. This antiparasitic used for roundworms and threadworms (pin worms) has been found to curb Covid viral replication (Panahi et. al. 2022). I had an intuitive hit about it, again for balancing the gut flora.
- Pavloxid. The FDA appoved this antiviral combination drug for use with acute Covid. Its effect on long Covid remains to be seen.

2. Herbal Antimicrobials
- Garlic. This antibiotic, anti-inflammatory can modulate the ACE-2 spike protein receptors (Abubakar et al. 2021).

> *I had many an intuitive hit for garlic and place it high on my list. Eat it raw every day (try two cloves three times a day) and mix it with honey for a "bait and bomb" effect on parasites. They come out for the sweet treat but get hit hard by the garlic bomb.*

- Resveratrol. Found in not just red wine and grapes but also Japanese knotweed. I found it to be an invaluable help for long Covid. I had many intuitive images of wine in a glass—that's resveratrol. It has been found to act against bacteria, fungi, cancerous tumors, and especially inflammation, among other things (Xiao et al. 2021). I place it high in my protocol.

- Cat's claw (*Uncaria tomentosa*) or Chinese cat's claw (*Uncaria rhynchophyllla*), which also modulates the immune system (Yepes-Pérez, Herrera-Calderon, and Quintero-Saumeth 2022). I had intuitive hits for it, expecially early on in my illness. See also Stephen Harrod Buhner's Covid-19 protocol (available on the website of the American Herbalists Guild) as he uses Chinese cat's claw for long Covid.

- Propolis, which is both antiviral and antihistamine, was found to interact with proteins from Covid-19 (Berretta et al. 2020) (Dilokthornsakul et al. 2022). I had a few "hits" for propolis and placed it in an herbal blend (see "Mold Drain Tincture" in appendix 4).

- Olive leaf extract/oleuropein, an antiviral and anti-inflammatory that may help manage Covid (Abdelgawad 2022).

- Wormwood (*Artemisia annua*). The tincture has proved effective against Covid (Zhou et al. 2021).

- Elderberry. Useful for treatment of viral illnesses (Wieland et al. 2021).

- Essential oils. Many have antiviral, anti-inflammatory, and immuno-modulatory effects effective that are helpful for acute Covid and long Covid (Asif et al. 2020). Try bay laurel, frankincense, juniper, oregano, rosemary, rosewood, and tea tree oil. Diffuse or nebulize these oils, or put a couple of drops on a hot washcloth and apply to the spine. With oregano, you can take a drop or two internally. I had quite a few intuitive hits for nebulizing rosemary in particular.

- Nicotiana (tobacco). Can help prevent spike proteins from binding to ACE-2 receptors (Mamedov et al. 2021). Nicotiana is toxic and very addictive and must be taken in very small amounts (as a tincture), but it is also a potent antibiotic and antiparasitic and great for mold (Ameya, Manilal, and Merdekios 2017; Rawat and Mali

2013). Some long-haulers have claimed that nicotine disrupts the spike proteins and use nicotine patches for this. I had many intuitive hits for tobacco and place it high on my list of important medicines. You can also try Hapé, or nasal tobacco. Treat tobacco as a powerful medicine only to be used respectfully and with prayer.

- Dragon's blood (*Croton lechleri*), a potent antiviral (Ubillas et al. 1994). I had an intuitive hit about this early on.
- South African geranium (*Pelargonium sidoides*), a potent antiviral effective against HIV (Helfer et al. 2014)

There are many other antimicrobial herbs that have been found to be quite effective, such as *Agaricus blazei, Lithospermum erythrorhizon, Lycium barbarum,* and others (Alhazmi et al. 2021).

3. Chemical Compounds and Supplements

- Peptides. Peptides have potent antibiotic, antiviral, anti-inflammatory, and immunomodulatory powers and can disrupt spike proteins (Khavinson et al. 2020). There are many on the market, but check out thymosin beta-4 (TB4), thymosin alpha-1 (TA1), LL-37, Selank, Cerebrolysin, and nicotinamide adenine dinucleotide (NAD) (Mahendran et al. 2020). I had many intuitive hits for NAD and found it to be very helpful. It is best administered as an IV, injectable peptide, or suppository.
- Colloidal silver. A potent antiviral and antibiotic (Jeremiah et al. 2020). I had so many images of silver spoons and silver pots, I consider colloidal silver as indispensable. Try a month on and then take a break for a week before resuming use; continuous long-term use can be detrimental.
- Food-grade hydrogen peroxide (2%), a powerful antiviral and antibiotic that has been found effective against Covid (Caruso et al. 2020). Caution: Use only food-grade 2% hydrogen peroxide, and just a few drops diluted in water for ingestion or, better, to nebulize. Can also be taken as an IV. I had many intuitive hits about this one.

- IV ozone. Found to be useful with Covid as an antiviral and anti-inflammatory (Cattel et al. 2021). Find a qualified practitioner to administer it. I did ten sessions of IV ozone and found it to be very helpful.
- Bee venom. Contains the peptide melittin, which has antiviral properties (Kasozi et al. 2020).

> *I had a powerful image of my daughter with a pacifier that said "bee venom" on it, so I trusted that and did some live bee sessions with an accupuncturist. I found it very helpful, and bee venom helped me over a bad hump.*

- Nitric oxide. This gas, which works like a free radical and can increase vasodilation and lower blood pressure, has been found to have an antimicrobial effect on Covid. (Adusumilli et al. 2020)
- Monolaurin (coconut-derived). It can inactivate viruses by disintegrating the viral envelope (Subroto and Indiarto 2020)
- Lysine. This amino acid impairs coronavirus replication (Müller et al. 2016).

CELLULAR HEALTH

This section on cellular health includes a broader list of remedies that can benefit mitochondria as well as antioxidants and free radicals that can clean up cellular debris, boost energy, and help with brain fog and general malaise.

1. Chemical Compounds
- Nitric oxide (see above)
- Nicotinamide adenine dinucleotide (NAD) (Miller, Wentzel, and Richards 2020)
- Methylene blue, a salt used as a dye and a medication, has been found helpful in Covid (Ghahestani et al. 2020)
- Palmitoylethanolamide (PEA), a chemical made from fat; also an anti-inflammatory (Keppel Hesselink, de Boer, and Witkamp 2013)

2. Supplements

- Niacin helps convert nutrients into energy, helps repair DNA, and exerts antioxidant effects. It is a precursor to NAD and a very important supplement for long-haul Covid. Many people use niacin as part of a vitamin "stack" (Nurek et al. 2021). The "Stamets Stack" combines niacin with lion's mane mushrooms and a microdose of psilocybin. Entire protocols revolve around niacin, with many believers.
- Glutathione, another important antioxidant places high on my list (Silvagno, Vernone, and Pescarmona 2020).
- IV vitamin C. Can help with fatigue, inflammation, and infections. I have met some long-haulers who claimed they healed completely using IV vitamin C. IV vitamin C was very helpful for me, especially when I was feeling horrible from histamine reactions.
- Vitamin E scavenges free radicals (Pizzorno 2014).
- N-acetylcysteine (NAC), an amino acid and natural antioxidant that is also essential for making the antioxidant glutathione (Shi and Puyo 2020). I found it helpful.
- Coenzyme Q10 and alpha-lipoic acid have been found helful for long-haul Covid when taken together (Barletta 2022).
- L-carnitine, an amino acid that transports fat to cells, can reduce long-haul Covid fatigue (Vaziri-Harami 2022).
- Theanine can improve mental function (Hidese et al. 2019).
- Specialized pro-resolving mediators (SPM) (Regidor 2020)
- Flavonoids, like luteolin (Theoharides et al. 2021) and those found in tart cherry (Chai et al. 2019)
- L-tryptophan—but with caution, as it can cause depression (Eroğlu, Eroğlu, and Güven 2021)
- Marine sponge, which is also anti-inflammatory (Alcaraz and Payá 2006)
- Policosanol, which also lowers cholesterol (Castaño et al. 2001)
- Shilajit (Winkler and Ghosh 2018)
- Melatonin, an anti-inflammatory and precurser to NRF2, can help with long Covid and with sleep (Mousavi et al. 2022). I had many intuitive hits for melatonin.

- NRF2, a protein that acts as a regulator of the body's antioxidant response, has been found helpful for long-haul Covid (Cuadrado et al. 2020).

GUT HELP

I covered a good deal on the gut in earlier chapters, but the products I found most helpful—in addition to prebiotics and probiotics such as Bifidobacterium, Akkermansia, *Baccilus subtilis,* and those found in buttermilk—were L-carnitine, butyrate, collagen, aloe vera, colostrum, opuntia, and inulin. Betaine HCL can improve gut function by helping to balance the gut flora and pH. It also has good antihistamine properties (Guilliams and Drake 2020). As described previously, I also had intuitive hits for killing bad gut bugs with amoxicillin, clindamycin, aspirin, and Coca-Cola, as well as mebendazole for parasites.

ESSENTIAL VITAMINS AND MINERALS

All the vitamins and minerals are important for health, but some are especially important for recovery from long Covid. To begin, I recommend getting a blood test to find any imbalances (especially ferritin and vitamin D) and to start taking a good liquid vitamin and mineral supplement. Also look into the bioavailability of supplements, as there are many different brands.

Keep in mind that much of your nutrition should come from foods. Turn to chicken soup for zinc and quercetin, for example, and to organ meats for iron and B vitamins, to Brazil nuts for selenium, and so on. Many of the intuitive hits I received were about foods I should eat. Of particular interest, note that a large study found that Covid patients had low levels of vitamin D and selenium (Im et al. 2020).

1. Vitamins
- Vitamin A, found in carrots and other vegetables
- Vitamin B$_1$ (thiamine)—some long-haulers megadose this for headaches

- Vitamin B_2 (riboflavin)—also comes as an IV and can be very helpful
- Vitamin B_3 (niacin)—some do megadosing protocols
- Vitamin B_6
- Vitamin B_8 (inositol)
- Vitamin B_9
- Vitamin B_{12}
- Vitamin C—some try megadosing
- Vitamin D—may or may not be helpful in long-haul (Townsend et al. 2021); my levels were always normal
- Vitamin E, a powerful antioxidant

2. Minerals

I had intuitive hits for all the following minerals:

- Phosphorus—I found supplementing with this mineral to be especially helpful
- Copper
- Magnesium—try glycinate
- Silica
- Selenium—try Brazil nuts
- Zinc
- Chloride
- Iron, if low—iron levels may also be high in long Covid patients, so be sure to have your ferritin levels checked (Kumar et al. 2021)

RELIEF FOR HEADACHES

1. Pharmaceuticals

- Nonsteroidal anti-inflammatory drugs (NSAIDs), like aspirin (which may also help with blood clots; Wijaya et al. 2021), ibuprofen, and acetaminophen

> *I had quite a few "hits" for aspirin not only for blood clots but also I believe it helps knock out bad guys in the gut from long Covid disbyosis.*

2. Natural Supplements

- Colostrum (see page 110)
- CBD oil and cannabis with THC, also a potent anti-inflammatory (Poudel et al. 2021)
- Salt water (Pogoda et al. 2016). I believe the sodium chloride is also helpful for breaking down spike proteins. Take ½ teaspoon in water twice a day. Also try supplements with redox versions of salt.
- Caffeine can reduce headaches and inflammation (Nowaczewska, Wiciński, and Kaźmierczak 2020).
- Lithium orotate, which is also helpful for depression and headaches (Sartori 1986)
- High-dose vitamin B_1 (theanine), which is also helpful for fatigue (Lubell 2021)

> *I had intuitive hits for CBD oil and cannabis by "seeing" a leaf of the marijuana plant. I often had hits for coffee but only a quarter-cup. I also had images of 9-volt batteries, which I connected to lithium!*

3. Homeopathics

I had many intuitive hits for most of the homeopathics below for headaches. They are inexpensive and can be very helpful. Try 30C or 200C.

- Natrum muriaticum
- Belladonna
- Iris
- Phosphoricum acidum
- Hepar sulphuris
- Sulphuricum acidum
- Cereus bonplandii
- Gelsemium
- Platinum
- Hyoscyamus niger (Witt, Lüdtke, and Willich 2010)

SLEEP HELP

1. Breathwork

Before going to sleep, try the Breath of Fire exercise (page 44) or just deep breathing—inhale for a count of four, hold for a count of four, exhale for a count of six (Lein 2021).

2. Herbs

- Valerian (Bent et al. 2006)
- Ashwagandha
- CBD oil (Shannon et al. 2019)

3. Other Options

- Magnesium glycinate, magnesium citrate, magnesium threonate
- Advil PM
- Melatonin, but don't take in combination with acetaminophen (Zhou et al. 2020)
- L-theanine, an amino acid helpful for relaxing the nervous system

BRAIN HEALTH: NEUROLOGICAL AND MEMORY SUPPORT

1. Herbs

Look for a good blend that includes the following or make your own blends:

- Ginkgo *(Ginkgo biloba)*
- Gotu kola
- St. John's wort
- Siberian ginseng *(Eleutherococcus senticosus)*
- Bacopa (Silveira et al. 2020)
- Skullcap
- Rosemary
- Passionflower
- Mint

2. Supplements

There are now many supplements and nootropics on the market that tout brain help. Many are a mix of the above herbs, amino acids, and other compounds. I found L-theanine helpful.

3. Remedies for Psychiatric Symptoms

This is an area where you should work with your doctor to address the causative issues and determine the right treatment. I found fluvoxamine very helpful, as it also works as an anti-inflammatory.

- SSRIs, such as sertraline (a.k.a. Zoloft) and fluvoxamine (Hamed and Hagag 2020; COVID-19 Early Treatment Fund, n.d.)
- St. John's wort

> I had a strong intuitive hit for fluvoxamine and used it for six months at a low dose (25 mg daily). I found that it helped take the "crazies" away and took the edge off my pain as well as helped my mood. I later used St. John's Wort, an herbal antidepressant. Do NOT take them together. I had a powerful vision where I saw a banner that said fluvoxamine/St. John's wort. To me that meant either or.

- Ketamine (Kera-Cov Research Group 2021)
- 5-HTP (Costa, Santos, and Branco 2020)
- Benzodiazepines (Ostuzzi et al. 2020)
- Homeopathic Stramonium
- Homeopathic Agaricus muscarius

BLOOD SUGAR MODULATORS

1. Pharmaceuticals

- Metformin, which is also helpful for modulating cytokine storms (Cory et al. 2021)

2. Herbs
- Opuntia (Hwang et al. 2017)
- Garlic

3. Supplements
- Chromium picolinate has been found to reduce blood glucose (Ali et al. 2011).
- Fulvic acid (Winkler and Ghosh 2018) and humic acid can significantly reduce blood glucose.

DEVELOP YOUR TREATMENT PROTOCOL

Clearly the lists above, though not comprehensive, are extensive. It can be quite overwhelming. They are meant as a guide, a way for you to see the possibilities, options, and categories of medicines. Keep in mind that the most effective treatments are those described in the earlier chapters, such as working with love and fire, meditations and breathwork, with the medicines as supplements to your recovery. Sometimes a long-hauler may find a magic bullet, but I can't say I did, and most won't. Most of us require all the tools in the medicine chest.

. . . .

Remember Your Most Important Medicine

Take three big breaths and then take a moment to reflect on the earlier chapters where we talk about love and fire as your most important medicines. The phrase "melt the disease in love" is what we want to hold paramount. Along with your attitudes and beliefs, your trust in your ability to heal will play play a huge part in your healing. Remember to return often to your love, fire, and breath, especially when you find yourself overwhelmed. I believe this is more powerful than any pill.

. . . .

When you are developing your protocol and determining which medications to take, I suggest choosing one or two from each category and utilizing the principles of rotation, synergy, and alchemy, as noted at the start of this chapter. There's no one right way, and your response may be different from another's response. This is where your intuition and a good functional medicine practitioner come into play. Keep in mind that from all of my research and intuitive work, I believe the main goal is to break down and flush out the lingering spike proteins and calm down or modulate the immune system.

Your simple daily protocol might look something like this:

1. Immunomodulating remedy like medicinal mushrooms or low-dose naltrexone (by prescription)
2. Spike protein breakdown remedy like homeopathic Silicea 30C or chlorine dioxide (**toxic**—proceed with extreme caution)
3. Monocyte receptor blocker like maraviroc (optional and by prescription only)
4. Anti-inflammatory like sea bucktorn oil
5. Antihistamine(s) that work for you, like Pepcid
6. Antimicrobial like garlic or monolaurin
7. Cellular rejuvenator like niacin or NAD (IV series administered by doctor)
8. Probiotics and gut builders like Bifidobacterium in kefir
9. Good daily vitamin and mineral supplements
10. Detoxification remedies like chlorella intermittently throughout

Be careful of overwhelming your body with a hodgepodge of pills. As mentioned earlier, I try to not take more than three remedies at a time and not more than five a day. Try tuning in to your body every morning and ask it what it needs. It is, after all, your body. Get to know what works and what doesn't.

MY TREATMENT PROTOCOL

My personal treatment protocol summary is provided in appendix 1.

OTHER PROTOCOLS

There are now so many protocols and recommended supplements. These were my favorite protocols:

1. Dr. Bruce Patterson's breakthrough highly successful treatment in dampening rogue monocytes. He uses CCR5 antagonist drugs like maraviroc and anibamine, statin drugs like atorvastatin, and ivermectin. You can find details and videos about this protocol online.
2. Master herbalist Stephen Harrod Buhner uses a protocol of herbs and supplements such as phosphatidylserine and choline, 5-HTP, tryptophan and Chinese cat's claw. You can find details on the website of the American Herbalists Guild.
3. The FLCCC protocol is available on the organization's website at Covidcriticalcare.com.
4. The website Mastcell360.com offers an in-depth discussion and corresponding protocol for mast cell activation syndrome and includes good information about mold, which are both issues with long Covid.

SUCCESS STORIES

Different long-haulers have had varying levels of success with the targets and remedies we discuss in this chapter. Some healed more quickly than others; some are still suffering. Here I've collected the treatment details from people who healed completely, listing what they consider their most important remedies.

Success #1
    Ivermectin
    Famotidine
    Statins

Positive attitude
Low-histamine diet
Omega-3s

Success #2

Microdosing psychedelic mushrooms, 0.5 gram daily, three days on,
one day off
Niacin (1 gram)
Lion's mane mushroom

Success #3

This was someone who did Dr. Bruce Patterson's protocol.

Maraviroc
Atorvastatin
Ivermectin

Success #4

Traditional Chinese medicine only

Success #5

Homeopathy only (with a classical homeopath) with the remedy
Sepia

Success #6

Long-term fasting (ten days)

Success #7

Low-dose prednisone
Ivermectin
Low-dose naltrexone

Success #8
    H1 and H2 antihistamines
    Fluvoxamine
    Ivermectin

Success #9
    Kambo
    Antihistamines

As you can see, there are many different paths out of the woods. You must find the one that leads you in the right direction. Perhaps you will pioneer a new path and show us the way.

10

✦ ✦ ✦

Calling on the Magic

Ceremony

WE ARE BLESSED TO HAVE MANY LIFE-FORMS surrounding us on this planet—plants, animals, and other organisms who can help us remember why we are here and where we came from. We are all intimately interconnected in this web of life. Since the beginning of time, people have been deeply connected to the natural world, relating to it as a source of food, shelter, clothing, and medicine and as a way to interface with their gods. It was once commonplace for people to know which herbs in their area could cure ailments and illnesses, or which animals they could pray to for healing, strength, or courage. Though most Western cultures have long forgotten these ways, we are fortunate enough to be alive during a time when many of these beliefs are reemerging to help humanity and our planet heal. We have the fantastic opportunity to reconnect with the hidden wisdom and power latent in the natural world by working with plants and animals for healing, just as our ancestors once did.*

Most indigenous cultures have some shamanic tradition where they connect with spirits as a direct interface with the divine. They reverently

---

*Much of the material in this chapter first appeared in *Liberating Yourself from Lyme*, chapters 14, "Plant and Animal Spirit Medicine," and 15, "The Great Mystery."

call upon these plants, animals, and the ancestors themselves as teachers and receive their wisdom and guidance in return (Jung 1968). While this concept may seem far-fetched to some, this ancient way of relating to Earth and her inhabitants dates back to our Paleolithic ancestors, and it lives on in some part of our consciousness, as certain animals are associated with symbolic meanings even to this day. In the United States the bald eagle is clearly recognized as a symbol of pride. Many people hold the grizzly bear as a symbol of protection. In visualizations and meditations, the image of a calm ocean is often called upon to create a feeling of peace in the body and mind. These are but a few examples of the way that our connection to nature is still intimately woven into our lives. I invite you to explore this a bit deeper by considering the ways in which you can learn from other plants and animals.

Many shamanic traditions believe that there are different realms of existence. We live in one realm, with what we see and perceive here, but upper and lower realms simultaneously exist, and the spirits and ancestors live there. In many traditions, it is possible to enter a trance-like state, where the veils between the worlds grow thin, through drumming, rattling, breathing, prayer, and working with plants. While we are in these realms, we have access to information and guidance we are otherwise unable to perceive or receive.

Who can help you face your fear by helping you find your inner fire and strength? Who can comfort you or stand by your side on this journey? Who can you call on for help?

SPIRIT ANIMALS

Call on animal helpers. Take a moment to contemplate what these animals have to offer, and see how they could be of help on your healing journey. You may have some unique animal to guide you, such as a tiger, bull, bear, wolf, eagle, or hawk. Try calling on the animals that resonate with you.

Mama bear can be there for you when the fear is overwhelming. Imagine a big grizzly or polar bear holding you like one of her cubs, fiercely protecting you from both seen and unseen forces. You can envision the grizzly claw carving out any disease. Bear claw is used in this way for shamanic purposes in many traditions. Fortunately we don't need to own a bear claw or eat bear gallbladder to receive the medicine of the bear. We can call on its spirit.

Tiger can be a great ally to help you awaken the fire in your belly and that sense of protection. The very image of a lion or tiger inspires respect, awe, and fierceness in most people. Those qualities live inside you as well, waiting to emerge and help you heal. Embody the tiger. Feel into what it would be like to chase down a gazelle at lightning speed, catch it, and eat it. This is a raw, primal part of ourselves that we seldom think about but has so much to offer us. By embodying the tiger or calling on the tiger spirit, you can chase down anything that wants to harm you and devour it. *Waking the Tiger,* by Steven Levine, is a landmark book that talks about awakening the inner tiger to move through trauma stored in the body into healing and a more profound sense of embodiment.

Owl would often come to me, and I found owl to be very wise, just like the stories of old. Owl arrived when I needed to make efficient decisions. In many Native American cultures, owl medicine can pierce through illusion or deception. It can achieve its goal with a single-pointed focus, which you can observe in the way owl hunts at night on silent wings. It can see as clear in the dark as in the light and thus is a wise ally. Call on owl medicine when you need to see clearly in a practical way or clear things away.

Use your creativity and imagination, as the possibilities here are limitless. Think about nature and observe her ways. Notice who eats what and the balance that is maintained through this circle of life and death. Eating something merely transforms that life-form, that food, into something else, liberating it as energy. Step into the ecology that you are. Try to transform Covid into something else in your alchemical pot, perhaps something you can use for your growth. Spike proteins are like little rocks. What animal would eat little rocks? Birds have a gizzard where they keep little rocks that help them digest food.

Call on imaginary birds to come and peck out the spike proteins.

Sometimes venomous or poisonous animals or plants, like rattle-snakes and black widow spiders, appear in our intuitive space. Consider that poisons might be what you need, in minute or even homeopathic amounts. Many resources can help you further explore connections with both plants and animals. The medicine card deck *The Discovery of Power through the Way of Animals,* by Jamie Sams and David Carson, is an excellent way to explore what can be learned from creatures that fly, crawl, run, and swim beside us on Earth.

PLANT SPIRIT MEDICINE

In the same way that most ancient cultures looked to animals for heal-ing, they also listened to plants as teachers and guides. Both modern-day indigenous cultures and an increasing number of herbalists and spiritual seekers hold the belief that plants have innate intelligence and a spirit that has much to teach us. Some cultures have ancient tradi-tions of working with plant medicines in shamanic ritual, taking a plant spirit into the body to receive the teachings and wisdom of those plants.

As previously discussed, in long Covid, the brain gets caught in a "limbic trauma loop" or a faulty default mode network (DMN). Meditation, neuroplasticity retraining, acupuncture, SSRIs, dissociative medicines, and psychedelic drugs can help us out of this loop. There are several plant teacher medicines of the psychedelic and psychoactive variety, including peyote (respect traditions here), San Pedro cactus, aya-huasca, iboga, and psilocybin mushrooms, as well as dissociative medi-cines like DMT (synthetic, 5-MeO-DMT, bufo). Kambo, the poisonous secretions from a tropical frog, though not a psychedelic, can be placed here, as can ketamine, though it is synthetic. These medicines, when used properly, can be of great benefit, and there are many stories of using them for healing from long Covid.

All of these medicines should be approached with the utmost respect and under the guidance of a trained shaman or guide. Many psychotherapists are now being trained to guide people on medicine journeys as a way to help them break through the stories of the past. The conscious mind is released or moved out of the way so that space can be held for the unconscious mind and stuck emotions to reveal themselves.

Psychedelic therapy has some benefit in modulating the immune system, reducing autoimmunity, and calming and resetting the immune system (Thompson and Szabo 2020). There are many methods and practitioners who can help you here. These medicines can also help us access deeper unfelt emotional issues and ancestral issues that may be dampening the immune system or causing a malfunction.

As medicines like ayahuasca are becoming more popular, let me impart a word of caution here and say that working with psychoactive plant medicine is not for everyone, and it is by no means necessary for healing. It is a powerful way to heal, but it is only for those who feel a strong calling to this work and have the constitution to sustain potentially destabilizing experiences. If you have bipolar disorder or any other psychiatric conditions (before developing long-haul Covid), the types of lessons offered by plant medicines can be challenging to handle and integrate.

Additionally, the legality of these plants vary from state to state, and local laws should be taken into consideration. These medicines can help us get down to the core self beneath the disease. They are just one of many ways to get there. I will say again that working with psychoactive plant spirit medicine is not a gentle path. It should only be explored if you are genuinely drawn to "walk into the fire" in this way and must be done with reverence and caution.

There are more gentle ways you can connect with plant spirits on your own, such as going out into nature and seeing which plants catch your attention. When you feel an energetic resonance with something, a medicine may be waiting to be discovered. The work (or fun) is to create a space to explore what that medicine is. I would suggest that you set aside some intentional time to be in nature and see what presents itself. It helps to breathe deeply and walk slowly when going on plant walks to quiet your mind and bring you into your sensing body. If you don't have access to a park or a forest, you can even do this in your backyard. Plants are everywhere, growing up out of cracks in the pavement, like dandelion and milk thistle. Wherever you are, scan the ground and see what plants jump out at you. Stop and sit beside the plant you noticed and see how it makes you feel. What does it remind you of? Does your body want that plant? Ask for the plants to come to help you.

An herbalist mentor of mine used to say that there are no weeds, only volunteers, and that one must pay extra close attention to the plants that volunteer their way into our lives and yards as they have things to teach us. The voices of plants do not speak as loudly as humans do, and we must quiet our minds enough to hear them. Often weeds are the most potent medicines as they have the resilience to sprout and take root without much nurturance or support.

Many books explore the connections to plant spirits and their innate intelligence, such as *The Secret Teachings of Plants,* by Stephen Harrod Buhner. This classic book explores the essence of who we are as people in our coevolving relationship with plants in a beautiful, poetic, and thought-provoking way. It is a must-read. Pam Montgomery's *Plant Spirit Healing* is another illuminating book, sharing a tremendous amount of wisdom and offering many exercises for different ways that you can step outside your rational mind. Open to a new way of relating to and learning from the green friends who are all around us. They have many gifts to share, even beyond purifying our air and soil, feeding our bellies, making our world more beautiful, and healing us with their medicine, all of which they do day in and out.

Please don't forget to make an offering to Earth and thank the plants and animals that have helped you if you call upon them for support.

MUSIC AND SOUND

Music is a powerful tool to reach the unconscious, to help us go in and access a deeper wisdom within ourselves, and can stimulate the brain for healing (Trimble and Hesdorffer 2017). I invite you to sing, dance, and pray at the same time. Put on some relaxing music, nature sounds, or James Brown; dance naked and shake it all out.

Making your own music and chanting is a fantastic way to access the liminal space, the place in between worlds.

✵ Music Exercise

Find a drum or a rattle and try to let go of any preconceived sense that you may have about not being musical or having rhythm. There is an African proverb that says, "If you can walk, you can dance. If you can talk, you can sing." The ability to express ourselves creatively lives within our bones. We need to get out of our heads and awaken to it. It is not hard to shake a rattle or play a simple repetitive beat on a small drum; you can use the rhythm of your heartbeat as a guide. Even just patting your hand on your leg will work. Most indigenous cultures use these methods to pray and enter trance states—they are as ancient as humanity. The goal is to enter a mental state that goes beyond the thinking mind and opens you up to the spirit realm, that place that exists just beyond the veil of what most people experience as reality.

Always begin by setting your intention with as much love as possible, calling in only the highest and most helpful guides for support. Close your eyes and notice your breath. Deepen your breath and start a beat with a rattle or drum. It can be helpful if you have a mantra or something to sing or chant repetitively, especially when beginning this type of journeying. Your chant could be as simple as "I am light, I am love, I am powerful, I am strong" or any phrase that resonates with you and your healing. Lighting candles or a fire can be a great addition.

As you drum and chant, continue to focus on deepening the breath and relaxing the body. Call for help from nature, inviting any plant or animal guides who have something to teach you to come forward. You can also call upon your inner guidance to provide insights into your healing. You may be amazed at what is revealed to you through this exercise. If thoughts or judgments emerge, just come back to your breath and stay focused on your intention. Try to sustain this for fifteen to twenty minutes. Always thank the spirit animals or plants that come to assist you, as your gratitude is part of what feeds and nourishes them.

Sound Healing

The world is vibrating. Some things slowly, some things quickly. We can use sound in the form of musical instruments like crystal bowls and gongs and even the sound of rain to help bring us back to balance.

The spike protein has a particular vibrational frequency. Just as a musical note or voice tone can shatter glass, so the right frequency might shatter it. Experiment with this, perhaps exploring tones or sounds you feel drawn to. Many practitioners today specialize in sound healing. There are also special sound devices used for this purpose.

Frequency Devices and Healing Machines

A Rife machine is a device designed by Royal Raymond Rife, an American inventor, to transmit a range of low-energy electromagnetic waves. The idea is that setting the device to the right frequency can cause disease molecules to excite and shatter. The phenomenon known as phase cancellation occurs when two signals of the same frequency are out of phase with each other, resulting in a net reduction in the overall level of the combined signal. If the two identical signals are 180 degrees out of phase (that is, 100 perent out of phase), they will cancel each other out if combined. This is in essence how the Rife machine and sound healing can work—by shattering and cancelling out the particular frequency of Covid.

There are many other specialty biofrequency and bioresonance devices that practitioners now use not only for healing but as diagnostic tools. Devices such as ZYTO or ASYRA, for instance, use a software program and the body's galvanic skin response to detect energetic imbalances in the body. My experience with these devices is that they can be great diagnostic tools but not necessarily good at clearing the disease.

There are other forms of vibrational healing as well, such as the use of electrical pulse devices like zappers, biophoton, color therapy, and therapies utilizing magnets. Again, there are specialists and practitioners who employ these methods. Many other cutting-edge technologies are just being discovered here; it may be the future of medicine.

LYING ON THE EARTH

Lying on the bare ground, or Earthing, has great benefit in helping us heal. Scientific studies have shown that walking barefoot or simply lying down in the grass, sand, or other ground surface can calm us down, increase oxygen efficiency, and decrease our heart rate (Chevalier et al. 2012). Even just imagining you are doing this can have benefit.

Try every day to get out into nature, and simply lie down, somewhere on the Earth. Imagine you are sinking down into the ground, and the Earth is taking the disease. Ask the trees and plants around you what will help you heal. The longer you can stay here, the better. Even better, take a camping trip, and sleep on the ground every night in your tent. The Earth can help.

CRYSTALS

I believe that quartz crystal and other gemstones can pull stagnant energy out of the body and that crystals can amplify your intentions to help you heal. They come from Earth and carry the wisdom of this planet, where they have lived for so many years. Quartz and other gemstones are essential allies in healing. Amethyst, which is a type of quartz, is particularly helpful for absorbing energy. Trust your guidance and check out some books on working with crystals if you are curious about this type of healing. The book *Love Is in the Earth,* by Melody, is a great place to start. I discovered that black tourmaline, selenite, and others can help with the overwhelming effects of electromagnetic frequencies, which are of particular concern with long Covid.

COLOR AND LIGHT HEALING

You can work with bringing colors or healing rays into your body during prayer or meditation for added strength and clarity. Imagine you are bringing these colors in through your crown chakra and down into your body, see the colors burn through and push out the disease through your tailbone into the Earth. Try "flashing" a flame or color in a particularly painful area. I found cobalt blue particularly useful to calm myself down. I used golden light and pure diamond white light to imagine clearing and cleansing my body. You can also work with the colors of the chakras: ruby red for the first chakra, tangerine orange for the second, a brilliant yellow like the sun for the third, emerald green for the fourth, brilliant sky blue for the fifth, indigo for the sixth, and a violet flame for the seventh (crown) chakra. If you feel drawn to color healing, there are practitioners who specifically work with color and healing. Also check out biophoton healing.

🌬 Violet Flame Meditation

Lie down or sit and make yourself comfortable. Close your eyes. Relax your body, relax your mind, and take three deep breaths. Now imagine a golden light from the heavens, the light of the brightest star, coming down from above though your crown and into your body, illuminating every cell. Imagine that light washing through you, down, and out your tailbone to the heart of the Earth. In the center of the Earth is a fiery core of lava, burning and transmuting all. Let the river of gold wash out the old immune cells, spike proteins, trash, and other "bugs," carrying them straight down to the center of the Earth. Open up and let it flow. Take some deep breaths. You can visualize bringing in the light with your inhalation, and washing it all out with your exhalation.

Once you have worked with the golden light, imagine a violet light, a violet flame, coursing through you in the same manner. It is a beautiful misty ray, like the top of the rainbow, a violet spritzer, calming, cooling, and washing out any leftover stagnancy, carrying it down to the center of the Earth. Let it go. Bless all the old cells; bless the new ones. Let the violet flame illuminate your entire body and energy field. *Blaze blaze blaze, consume consume consume, transmute transmute transmute.* Take some deep breaths.

Now, with the same process, bring in a cobalt blue energy, a crystalline, icy, cooling blue. Let it mist through you, calming, cooling, stilling, healing, and chilling your nervous system. Bathe your amygdala and limbic system in the center of your brain. It is an icy cobalt blue mountain lake. Breathe slow and deep. Try to feel the color, become the color, become the stillness of the lake.

When you are ready, open your eyes and thank yourself and any angels who assisted you.

FOCUS AND DISCIPLINE

We have looked at many ways and angles to work with long-haul Covid, but in my experience the most important place to return to is the awareness that you are not a disease. Your spirit is made of unconditional love and is incredibly powerful. The power of your spirit can overcome this illness as it exists in the body. Make that your mantra. Sing, chant, dance, and pray to awaken and nourish what you are: love and fire. Find the right medicines that your own body is telling you you need. Try to take on the mind of an athlete—believing that you are going to win, no matter how many times you have to start the race over.

It takes determination, focus, and discipline. Return to these empowering qualities again and again. Try to focus on what's right. Sometimes we are so busy focusing on what's bad or what's not right that we forget the parts of us that are just fine. Instead, try looking at what's right and spreading it around. Your awareness is an integral part of creating your reality. Perhaps you can focus on the good things in your life that bring you joy and the people that you love.

THE CALL FOR HELP

It's so important to ask for help, support, and assistance. Ask for help from your community. Being in pain all the time is annoying. In a culture that is connected through technology and social media, we can forget about the simplicity of physical contact and support at times. On the most basic level we need each other to survive. Long-haul Covid patients can tend toward isolation when they are sick. There can be the sense that no one else knows what we are going through or could understand, or we are too embarrassed to be seen and not functioning adequately. A common reaction I would encounter was "You're *still* sick?"

Long Covid is hard to explain to people who do not understand it. This disease demands that we reach out for help and look toward our community to support us as we come back into balance. It is a real opportunity for growth on many levels for all people involved. If you are an independent person or a caregiver yourself, you have to allow your friends to show up for you. There are many support groups online with people dealing with the same symptoms. Together we can find the solutions, share them, and climb out.

Many times when I was totally broken and delirious, I called for help. Not only to those seen but also to those unseen. When you call on Ascended Masters and helper angels (Jesus, Mother Mary, St. Germain, Quan Yin, Archangel Michael, and so on), nature spirits and guides, they will come. Place yourself in a humble place, pour out your love, and call for help and listen for guidance. They may send you light in the form of a color; work with bringing that in. Many benevolent beings are here to help. Some of the intuitive guidance I received came from them. Trust those you love and make the call, then listen for their guidance.

Call on your friends to do a synchronized prayer for you over social media. Have everyone pray for your healing at a set time for a few minutes or so. Better yet, have some friends come over and lay their hands on you, just sending love.

Don't hesitate to find a good doctor or healer who specializes in long-haul Covid, someone who really gets it and knows how to treat it.

A functional or integrative medicine practitioner may be best, because you're going to need a full spectrum of options.

TAKING BACK THE POWER

I spent far too much money on doctors, healers, and pills in my journey with long Covid, to a point where I was obsessing about the illness and healing. I ended up with conflicting pills, protocols, stories, diagnoses, and so on. If you have that same experience, there may come a time when not only can you simply not afford it anymore, but you have to let the "diagnosis" and your association with it go. If you begin to relate to yourself as someone who is always sick or a "long-hauler," beware the victim mentality. Ask yourself if you are ready to be done being sick. Consider what it would look like to stop identifying as someone who is sick with long Covid. Consider focusing on what is right with your body instead of what is wrong. It is easy to get so caught up in thinking about disease that we miss out on what we love. I am sharing this from personal experience.

Forget about how you were in the past. Make a new normal and start from where you are. This doesn't mean you shouldn't seek help; it means consider letting go of the story and the obsession with needing to heal. You're going to have to trust that there will be an end point. It just may take time. Consider whether there is a part of you that *is* healed, a place that is not sick. Access that place as much as you can, let go of the story of why, and focus on what is. Use your intuition to help guide you how to heal. What's your body saying? It is your body, after all.

Have fun and laugh. Do what you love: sing, dance, make art, make love, go jump in the river, reach out to others who are suffering more than you, and most of all, trust love.

Laughter
Sometimes laughter can be incredibly healing, even in the most dire of situations. Be sure to make others laugh, watch great comedians, be silly, and even make fun of the disease and yourself. When we laugh, suddenly

things aren't so serious, and we can let go of some heaviness. Surprisingly, we can sometimes come back to an issue or problem with greater clarity. I never trust a teacher or guru who doesn't make me laugh.

What Do You Love to Do?

We can spend days and days focused on healing, looking at pills and remedies, doctors' appointments, books, methods, and so on. We may spend all day thinking about our disease and what do about it. Or we may be focused on the pain we are in, constantly fretting and moaning about it. Yes, pain and suffering suck, but sometimes not focusing on it is when we can really heal. I had this vision of myself as an old man, alone and surrounded by piles of manuscripts and scientific research on Covid and other diseases. I was staring at a computer looking for answers, going deep down some wormhole. Yuck. This image was so nauseating to me. Is this what I want? Heck no. My deepest passion is music and art. Then I had a dream where I was playing music on a big stage, and I woke up with a feeling of passion, of deep fire and desire. Yes! This is what I want.

So focus on what you love and the people you love. Distract yourself from the suffering. Make art. Pick up a paintbrush, create a junk sculpture in the backyard, call up that person, get voice lessons. You get the idea. Stay focused on what you love, even if you're doing it from your bed.

EMBODIMENT

I have met many people with long-haul Covid who struggle with stuck emotions: they feel disconnected, dissatisfied, and disaffected. Burying emotional pain is a form of psychological or spiritual bypass, and it leads to disembodiment—we are not fully present in our body or our lives. Having felt this way before myself, I believe that it is precisely this disembodiment or nonpresence that can make us more susceptible to sickness and less able to heal.

As we discussed in chapter 4, processing emotional issues and unsticking stuck feelings is an important part of supporting our energetic immunity. Taking responsibility for what is not working in our life is the first step to healing.

DISEASE AS A TEACHER

You need courage to be here, to heal your wounds, even if you don't want to. Sometimes the way out is through the pain. You are not alone, and realizing that in and of itself helps calm pain. There are allies, doctors, and healers supporting you on this path of healing, and it can become a path of awakening if our journey teaches us to embrace stronger boundaries, greater love, and full embodiment.

If we can see disease as a teacher, we may transform our perspective on what disease is. Doing so opens an exploration into our impermanence, the truth that someday we will have to let go of these bodies. What does acknowledgment of impermanence teach us? The answers are ours to discover through realizations of the mysteries.

Consider praying for and blessing the success and joy of others, even those you are jealous of or dislike. Recall the lines from the poem cited in chapter 2: *Forgive yourself from the past. Support your immune system to do its task.*

Allow any wall around your heart to fall; let your heart be a conduit that gives and receives only love. Keep it open, you will heal quicker.

What about children who have long haul? Do they have all the issues outlined in this book, too? Perhaps there are no underlying issues, and the child is just sick. Perhaps there are ancestral or genetic issues that have been passed on to the child. Perhaps not. These are questions that you may ask as a parent of a sick child. Then the parent becomes the guardian, the healer, the liberator.

Children may heal faster and more easily because their immune systems are usually less stressed and their circulation is better, bringing medicines and immune factors through the bloodstream more efficiently than an adult would. Consider being more childlike in your physical, mental, and spiritual behavior as part of your healing. See what it feels like to lighten up, to play and flow more.

Love like there's no tomorrow because there might not be.

Each moment is a new opportunity to look deep inside. What do you have to let go of? Whose voice are you listening to: fear or love? It's important to have a sense of curiosity when you ask these questions. Notice if your inner monologue goes to judgment, and see if you can invite the voice of compassion. Treat yourself like you would treat a small child who is still learning. It's only through becoming aware of our issues that we can do the work needed to transform them. It begins with choosing to listen to the voice of love, no matter what. It also takes verifying any intuitive information that you receive with love. Hold fast and trust love as if it were your last day on Earth.

TIME

In the end, healing from long Covid just may take time. A lot of time. You will get there. The spike proteins will flush out, the old autoantibodies will die off, and your body will return to normal. Your immune system can restore itself. You just may have to be patient. It's a marathon, not a sprint. One step at a time.

DEATH

Ultimately, healing is a mystery. Some people heal, and others struggle. Some are not ready or do not want to heal. Grace and miracles come into play here more than most of us might think. Many things are yet to be discovered in this universe. The healthiest person might die tomorrow, and the sickest person might have a miracle today. We never really know what's coming. What would you do today if you were not here tomorrow? How would you live fully in this precious moment? Who would you make peace with? What would you forgive yourself for? The power is in you. Each day is an opportunity for love. Every single day holds the chance to start fresh, so seize the moment.

The Heisenberg uncertainty principle in physics says: "You can never really know where an electron is at any given time; it, therefore, does not have a perfect order" (Zalta 2006). The perfection of the universe is in the imperfection of the world as it seeks to know itself. The universe has a tendency toward order and health. I believe, as many do, that chaos and darkness serve their purpose, prompting us to come back to love with an even stronger resolve.

We may die tomorrow. How afraid of death are we? With diseases we learn to die again and again metaphorically. With this illness we may even face our actual death, or think, as I did, that we are going to die. The more that we can accept and surrender to the energy of death as part of the cycle that is existence, the more we can learn to rest in it. *Death is birth.* Through practice we can even find peace with death, knowing that it will lead to rebirth just as winter is always followed by spring. Knowing that we are part of something greater, as it is mirrored in the cycles of Earth, I believe we can get to a place beyond fear where we welcome death.

What practices help us to let go? What are we most afraid of when we think about the idea of death? How can we explore these ideas with openness and curiosity, rather than fear and terror? What can our disease teach us? How can we learn from long-haul Covid?

Choosing to say yes to disease as our teacher, rather than allowing ourselves to become the victim, is ultimately choosing love over fear. When we make a conscious choice of trusting love, regardless of what is happening, we become a reflection of a love that is much greater than our sense of self. It calls us first to recognize and then surrender to that greater love or divinity as it moves through us. Sometimes it can happen in unexpected or undesirable ways. Therein lies the journey: healing the suffering of the body and mind with the love of our spirit, which I believe is the truth of who we are. It is the spark of love that lights the fire of our healing, starting from inside and radiating out.

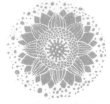

✦ ✦ ✦

Why Covid?

Moving toward a Collective Healing

THERE HAS BEEN MUCH SPECULATION on the origin of Covid-19. The virus was thought to have originated in Wuhan, China, as a spillover infection from animals to humans in December 2019, or possibly earlier. Or perhaps it originated in a laboratory, with scientists amplifying the potency of the virus as part of their research. Or perhaps it was created as a bioweapon. Theories abound, the debate continues, and we may never definitively know.

What I believe has broader implications. Shortly after I was sick with Covid, while meditating, I "heard" the phrase *upset Earth,* loud and clear. It got me thinking about the idea of an upset Earth, or that Earth has a consciousness and this Gaian awareness was upset. Is this possible? Why would the Earth be angry?

The global loss of biodiversity just in the past hundred years is astounding. If the current rate of deforestation continues linearly, tropical forests will be gone in two hundred years, with a concurrent animal and insect species extinction rate greater than that of four of the five previous mass extinctions on this planet (Giam 2017). A 2020 report from the World Wildlife Fund estimates that we lost two-thirds of the world's wildlife in the past fifty years. At the same time, even conservative estimates place species extinction rates at two hundred to two thousand species a year (World Wildlife Fund n.d.). Pollution from fossil fuels, climate change, environmental degradation, agricultural monoculture, and much more all lead to an Earth in peril. Studies even show that deforestation and loss of wildlife cause an increase in rates of infectious disease. And who is the cause? Humans, of course.

Later on in my illness, I was feeling into my brain fire and "saw" clear images of dry, cracked mud and giant freshly cut tree stumps. It dawned on me that the pain I was feeling was a reflection of what's happening to the Earth. My painful scorching daily headaches, the brain fire, the malaise, the confusion—is this what Earth is feeling? Is this what species that are going extinct feel? Is it possible that the natural world around us—Earth and all its species—feels this pain on a collective level? I would say yes, absolutely.

What if Earth sent out Covid? What better way to slow us down? To stop our unsustainable behavior? If I were the planet, a global pandemic sounds like a good way to carry this out. Upset Earth indeed. It reminds me of poking a stick into a beehive, and all the hot little angry creatures come pouring out to inflict pain on us.

So, then, in my opinion, Covid is a symptom of something much greater, of a planetary system fallen out of balance, a reflection of what Earth is experiencing now. From this perspective, Covid is a result of ecological instability, and we humans are responsible for it. Many scientists have come to the same conclusion (Quinney 2020).

THE COLLECTIVE HEALING

If we acknowledge that Earth is out of balance, then what is the healing? Everything we have explored in this book: feeding the inner fire, calming the overreactive immune system, detoxifying, resting, slowing down, simplifying, looking inward, practicing forgiveness, focusing on what's important, what we love, what really matters. All of this affects the planet.

We might even say that as long as we're practicing forgiveness, we owe Earth an apology. Remember how, during the height of the pandemic, when so much of the human population was forced to stay home, air pollution was greatly reduced and animals appeared in the streets? Regulation, restoration, and regeneration are necessary for new neural connections, new networks of symbiosis, more diversity, and stronger immune systems, both for us and for Earth. And we all might benefit from a practice of asking Earth for forgiveness and making offerings to the world. How can we make offerings to help heal the planet? Consider that simply planting a tree, composting, or planting a garden can be a type of offering back to the Earth. (Check out *Braiding Sweetgrass,* by Robin Kimmer, for a deeper dive into the concept of forgiveness and offerings to the Earth.)

How can we be more mindful of our effect on the planet? Perhaps we can start by living more simply. Do we really need every last product our culture tells us we do? We might ask whether we really need each new thing, where it came from, who or what it affected, where it will go when we're done with it, and what might be the effect of its disposal. In my opinion, true abundance is not material but energetic. Our lives are fulfilling when our spirits, not our homes, are full.

Take only what you need, share, and keep the Earth in mind.

Consider that our own healing reflects back to Earth, that our lives are very much entwined with a greater consciousness, a greater love, a collective healing.

ACCEPTANCE

Sometimes we don't heal the way we want to, sometimes we die, sometimes we just can't do it yet. The Earth may become more polluted and we will certainly lose more species. Consider accepting these outcomes. We will all die someday anyways. Consider letting go and surrendering to what is. Consider becoming the eye of a hurricane. Consider being grateful for what we do have now, and focusing on what's working and what's positive now, rather than focusing on what's wrong, the despair of the future, and the victimhood. We can then work toward a potentiality of health and ecology against seeming odds.

Don't give up. Trust love always. It will heal you.

With Covid—as with any "enemy"—thank it, bless it, burn it.

Appendices

∽∾∽

Note: I designed the following exercises and remedies based on my intuitive knowledge and experiences from over the years. They are what worked for me. Please consult with a doctor, herbalist, or homeopath for proper guidance and dosages.

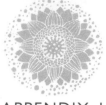

✦ ✦ ✦

Treatment
Protocol Summary

IN THE FOLLOWING CHART YOU WILL FIND my personal treatment protocol—derived from intuition and a lot of research. This is what worked for *my* body. I did not take more than five remedies a day or three at a time, and no more than eight in a week. I never used more than two spike protein breakdown remedies at a time. I rotated remedies in and out. I looked for synergy and alchemy, and I took breaks.

***Always consult with a doctor before beginning
your own treatment protocol.***

For more information see the protocols on the FLCCC website (https://covid19criticalcare.com/treatment-protocols) and my personal site, VirMcCoyHealth.com.

REMEDY FUNCTION (choose one or two from each category)	TYPE	PRODUCT	DOSAGE	NOTES
Immune Support and Modulation	Pharmaceuticals (optional)	Low-dose naltrexone	As directed	By prescription only; see also FLCCC protocol
	Herbs	Reishi, turkey tail, chaga, lion's mane	1 Tbsp of each as powders, 3x a day	I mixed these together in my "Immune-Boosting Mushroom Milk" (see appendix 4)
	Other Compounds	Ashwaganda	2 (1 ml-) droppersful a day or 1 Tbsp powder	
		Colostrum	2 heaping Tbsp., 3x a day	Also try lactoferrin
		IVIg	As directed	By prescription only
	Psychedelics	Psychedelic mushrooms	Microdose for 2 days on, 1 off for a month	Check the legality in your state or country; can rotate with microdosing others such as San Pedro cactus and LSD
Spike Protein Breakdown	Detergents	Chlorine dioxide	1–5 drops diluted, 2x a day	*Toxic*—proceed with extreme caution
		Sodium hydroxide (lye)	1–5 drops diluted and with fat, 2x a day	*Toxic*—proceed with extreme caution
		Sodium Chloride (salt)	½ tsp. diluted, 2x a day	Can be purgative in large amounts
	Saponins	Agave leaf tincture	1–5 drops diluted, 2x a day	*Toxic*—proceed with extreme caution; rotate with other saponins
		Licorice tincture	1 ml dropperful, 2x a day	Rotate with other saponins
		Horse chestnut tincture	1 ml dropperful, 2x a day	Rotate with other saponins

REMEDY FUNCTION *(choose one or two from each category)*	TYPE	PRODUCT	DOSAGE	NOTES
Spike Protein Breakdown *(continued)*	Enzymes	Nattokinase	Up to gut tolerance, 2x a day on empty stomach	
		Lumbrokinase	Up to gut tolerance, 2x a day on empty stomach	
		Protease	Up to gut tolerance, 2x a day on empty stomach	
	Homeopathics	Silicea 30C	2–3 pellets, 2–3x a day	Take for one week, then shift to the next homeopathic
		Graphites 30C	2–3 pellets, 2–3x a day	Take for one week, then shift to the next homeopathic
		Petroleum 30C	2–3 pellets, 2–3x a day	Take for one week, then shift to the next homeopathic
		China 30C	2–3 pellets, 2–3x a day	Take for one week, then shift to the next homeopathic
		Thuja 30C	2–3 pellets, 2–3x a day	Take for one week, then shift to the next homeopathic
	Acids	Shikimic (pine needles, star anise, fennel)	As tea	Make your own tea blends
		Fulvic and humic acid	As tea or tincture, as directed	

REMEDY FUNCTION (choose one or two from each category)	TYPE	PRODUCT	DOSAGE	NOTES
Spike Protein Breakdown (continued)	Acids (continued)	Nicotinic acid (niacin)	100 mg a day; increase dosage until flush (hot rash-like sensation), then reduce as needed so dosage results in just slight flush	Can also megadose (see Dmitry Kats protocol); but use caution
	Alcohol	Mescal	Try 2 shots, 2x a week	May cause histamine reaction
		Wine	Try 2 glasses, 2x a week	May cause histamine reaction
	Terpenes	Turpentine	1–3 drops in a glass of water, 2x a day	*Toxic*—proceed with extreme caution
Monocyte Receptor Blockers (Optional Pharmaceuticals)	ACE-2 Blockers	Ivermectin	As directed by doctor	By prescription only; see also FLCCC protocol
		Hydroxychloroquine	As directed	By prescription only; see also FLCCC protocol
	CCR5 Blockers	Maraviroc	As directed	By prescription only; see also FLCCC protocol
	Fractalkine Blockers	Statins	As directed	By prescription only; see also FLCCC protocol
Anti-inflammatories	Pharmaceuticals	Aspirin and other NSAIDS	81 mg a day or as directed	See also FLCCC protocol
		Fluvoxamine	As directed	By prescription only; see also FLCCC protocol
	Steroids	Prednisone	As directed	By prescription only

REMEDY FUNCTION (choose one or two from each category)	TYPE	PRODUCT	DOSAGE	NOTES
Anti-inflammatories (continued)	Oils	Black currant seed oil	As much as you like	Hot is best
		Black seed (Nigella sativa) oil	As much as you like	Hot is best
		Sea buckthorn oil	As much as you like	Hot is best
		Olive oil	As much as you like	Hot is best
		Avocado oil	As much as you like	Hot is best
		Fish oil (omega-3)	As much as you like	Hot is best
	Herbs/ Supplements	Resveratrol (Japanese knotweed)	1,000 mg a day	Try bioavailable forms
		CBD oil	1–2 (ml) droppersful, as needed	
		Fresh turmeric or curcumin	1 finger a day or as directed	Mix with milk and black pepper
		Boswellia	Essential oil or supplement; follow manufacturer's instructions	
	Peptides	BPC-157, thymosin alpha-1, or hecogenin	As directed	Prescription only injection
Antihistamines and Mast Cell Stabilizers	Pharmaceuticals	H1—cetirizine	2x a day or as directed	Mix and match with H2 antihistamine
		H2—famotadine (Pepcid, etc.)	2x a day or as directed	
		Ketotifen	As directed	By prescription only
		Cromolyn sodium	As directed	By prescription only
	Natural Antihistamines	Quercetin	500 mg, 2x a day	Also try with bromelain, nettles
		Skullcap	1–2 (ml) droppersfull a day	Try with Pepcid

REMEDY FUNCTION (choose one or two from each category)	TYPE	PRODUCT	DOSAGE	NOTES
Antihistamines and Mast Cell Stabilizers (*continued*)	Natural Antihistamines (*continued*)	Ephedra	1 ml dropperful of tincture, 2x a day	Ephedra is illegal in the United States; synthetic ephedrine is available by prescription
	Other Compounds	Baking soda (sodium bicarbonate)	½ tsp. in glass of water, 2x a day	
		Vitamin C	1,500 mg, 2x a day	Can add to baking soda drink with ¼ tsp. salt; IV vitamin C is also an option
		Bee venom	10 stings a week	Work with a practitioner
	Homeopathics	Histaminum, Apis, or Rhus toxicodendron	2–3 pellets a day	Work with a homeopath
Antimicrobials	Western Pharmaceuticals (Antiparasitics)	Ivermectin	As directed by doctor	By prescription only
		Hydroxychloroquine	As directed	By prescription only
		Mebendazole	As directed	By prescription only for parasites
	Herbal Antimicrobials	Garlic	6 cloves a day	
		Resveratrol (Japanese knotweed)	1,000 mg, 2x a day	Try bioavailable forms
		Propolis	1 ml dropperful, 3x a day	Honey as well
		Essential oils (e.g., oregano, rosemary)	Diffuse or nebulize daily	
		Nicotiana tincture	1–4 drops a day	*Toxic*—proceed with extreme caution
	Chemical Compounds and Supplements	Colloidal silver	2 (1 ml-) droppersful a day for one month, then take a week off	Continuous long-term use can be detrimental

REMEDY FUNCTION (choose one or two from each category)	TYPE	PRODUCT	DOSAGE	NOTES
Antimicrobials (*continued*)	Chemical Compounds and Supplements (*continued*)	Hydrogen peroxide	A few drops (food grade 2%) in a glass of water or nebulized	Can also be administered as an IV (by a doctor)
		IV ozone	As directed	Administered by doctor
		Monolaurin	2 capsules a day or as directed	Can be taken orally, as injectable peptide, IV, or suppository
Cellular Health	Compounds	NAD	As directed	
	Supplements	Niacin	100 mg a day; increase dosage until flush (hot rash-like sensation), then reduce as needed so dosage results in just slight flush	See also Dmitry Kats protocol; use caution
		Glutathione	Nebulize	
		IV vitamin C	As directed	Administered by doctor
		Vitamin E	Manufacturer's suggested dosage	
		NAC	700 mg a day or manufacturer's suggested dosage	
Gut Help		Prebiotics (try chicory)	Manufacturer's suggested dosage	
		Probiotics high in Bifidobacterium and *Bacillus subtilis*	Manufacturer's suggested dosage	Get a gut microbiome test to determine which probiotics in particular you may need to supplement
		L-Carnitine	500–2000 mg or manufacturer's suggested dosage	

REMEDY FUNCTION (choose one or two from each category)	TYPE	PRODUCT	DOSAGE	NOTES
Gut Help (continued)		Butyrate	150–300 mg a day or manufacturer's suggested dosage	
		Aloe vera	Manufacturer's suggested dosage	
		Betaine HCL	Manufacturer's suggested dosage	Increase dosage slowly
		Amoxicillin	As directed	May help kill bad gut bugs; by prescription only
		Aspirin	81 mg a day or manufacturer's suggested dosage	May help kill bad gut bugs; see also FLCCC protocol
Essential Vitamins and Minerals	Vitamins	Vitamins A, B_1, B_2, B_3, B_6, B_8, B_9, B_{12}, C, D, E	Find a good blend and use as directed	High doses of B_1, B_2, and B_3 may also be indicated. See your doctor about IV B_2
	Minerals	Phosphorus, copper, magnesium, selenium, zinc—and iron *only if levels are low*	Find a good liquid blend and use as directed	
Detoxification (see chapter 7)	Herbs for Lymphatic Drainage	Ocotillo tincture	1–3 droppersful a day or manufacturer's suggested dosage	Detox once a week or as needed
		Red root (ceanothus) tincture	1–3 droppersful a day or manufacturer's suggested dosage	
	Detoxifying Heavy Metals	Chlorella	2 scoops or manufacturer's suggested dosage	Detox once a week or as needed; look for a good blend of these with clay and other herbs—also for mopping up mold
		Zeolite clays	Manufacturer's suggested dosage	
		Charcoal	Manufacturer's suggested dosage	
		Wheatgrass	Fresh or powder; the more the better	

REMEDY FUNCTION (choose one or two from each category)	TYPE	PRODUCT	DOSAGE	NOTES
Detoxification (continued) (see chapter 7)	Herbs for Body Detoxification	*Mucuna pruriens* (velvet bean) powder	Manufacturer's suggested dosage	Detox once a week or as needed
	Detox Baths	Personalized blend	1–2 cups baking soda, 1–2 cups Epsom salts, 1 cup bentonite clay, 1 cup borax; soak for 20 minutes once a week	
Ceremony (optional; see chapter 10)	Plant Spirit Medicine	Various dissociative medicines	As directed	Work with qualified shaman or practitioner only
Relief for Headaches (as/if needed)	Pharmaceuticals	NSAIDs (aspirin, ibuprofen, acetaminophen)	As needed; follow manufacturer's instructions	
	Natural Supplements	Lithium ororate	Manufacturer's suggested dosage	
	Homeopathics	Try Iris, Belladonna, Sulphuricum acidum	1–3 pellets 2–3x a day as needed	Work with a homeopath
Sleep Help (as/if needed)	Herbs	CBD oil	Manufacturer's suggested dosage	
	Other Options	Melatonin	Manufacturer's suggested dosage	Do not take in combination with acetaminophen
Brain Health (as/if needed)	Remedies for Psychiatric Symptoms	SSRIs (e.g., Fluvoxamine)	As directed	By prescription only
		St. John's wort	1–3 droppersful or manufacturer's suggested dosage	Do not take with SSRIs (such as fluvoxamine); best taken away from other herbs
		5-HTP	Manufacturer's suggested dosage	
Blood Sugar Modulators (as/if needed)	Pharmaceuticals	Metformin	As directed	By prescription only
	Herbs	Opuntia cactus	Eat fresh as desired	
	Supplements	Chromium picolinate	50–200 mcg a day or manufacturer's suggested dosage	

Important Daily Practices and Reminders

- Develop your medical intuition
- Work with a good functional or integrative practitioner
- Rest, reduce stress, meditate, pray, take sunset walks, spend time in nature
- Remove yourself from moldy environments
- Reduce screen time and EMF exposure
- Breathwork—Breath of Fire, Buteyko Breathing, Wim Hof Method
- Detox—sweat in a sauna; perform lymphatic movement exercises
- Hydrate—drink a gallon of water a day (try bubbly waters and ice water along with ice baths, cold showers, dips in an icy river, etc.)
- Fasting, intermittent fasting, and juicing (apples, ginger, celery, turmeric)
- Low-histamine ketogenic diet
- Vagus nerve stimulation, neuroplasticity retraining, neurogenesis, brain exercises
- Gentle and gradual physical exercise—yoga, hot yoga, weights, jumping, jogging

APPENDIX 2

+ + +

Fire Love Loop Exercise

WE MUST CULTIVATE A FIRE IN THE BELLY and love for ourselves in order to bring about healing.

The Fire Love Loop exercise contains three parts. The first part is a modified microcosmic orbit. (See Mantak Chia's excellent book *Awaken Healing Light* for further study, or look for my self-help videos on YouTube.) This part of the exercise is about generating fire and love, which you will apply toward freeing yourself from long Covid (or other disease) in parts two and three. For a visual, please go to YouTube and look up "Vir McCoy, Fire Love Loop Breathing Technique."

To get the fire in your belly started, we are going to use the analogy of a car engine. Imagine that the liver is an oil tank with fuel oil and the gallbladder is the regulator with a valve. The fuel pump will squirt fuel oil onto the spark plug located at the solar plexus, about three fingers' width below your belly button, where oxygen from your breath will help ignite a fire and get your engine going. Once the engine is running and the fire is burning in the belly, we will bring the fire up the spine (the transmission) to the head and then bring it back down the front of the body through the heart (the radiator), cooling the energy, back through the belly, and down out the tailbone (the exhaust). From the side it will look like a large loop.

It is helpful to do this exercise while gazing at a fire or a candle; the best time to do it is during sunset or sunrise.

PART I: THE FIRE LOVE GENERATOR

1. Find a quiet place and sit upright, either cross-legged on the floor or in a chair, or lie on your back.

2. To warm up, gently rock the lower part of your body back and forth (like a cat stretch in yoga, but not as intense). As your back arches forward, inhale, and as your back arches backward, exhale. This loosens up the lower spine and gets the breath ready. Do this sixty times. Then rest for a moment and focus on your upper body.

3. Place the tips of your fingers on the outsides of your shoulders to create wings. Begin to flap them back and forth like butterfly wings, opening your chest and coming forward, bringing your elbows toward each other at the back. Then collapse your chest and bring your elbows together at the front of your body. This warms the upper body. Notice the natural exhalation as your elbows come together at the front of your body, and the inhalation as they come back. Do this sixty times. Rest.

4. Breathe in and out slowly from your belly. Start by exhaling all your air and flattening your belly. Sit up straight. Now bring your inhalation as low into your belly as you can so that on the inhalation your belly becomes a big balloon. Then again, on exhalation, bring your abdominal muscles tight toward your back as much as you can. Continue this slow belly breathing for fifteen breaths. As you are doing this, begin to expand on the breath by exaggerating the movement of the lower part of your body back and forth with the inhalation and exhalation (again, like a cat stretch, where your back arches forward on the inhale and back on the exhale).

5. As you're doing this, imagine and feel with your senses, and focus with your mind on a spot just below your navel and toward the back of the spine where your spark plug or little fire is. Focus the heat you are creating in this hot spot. This is the center of inner fire, chi, or tan tien. You might also imagine you are going to make a fire in this spot by spinning a stick back and forth on a little bit of

tinder. See it burst into flames and create a fire in your inner stove. Try to feel the heat.

6. Touch your thumbs and the tips of all your fingers together and place them over your fire center, creating a triangle shape. These are liver mudras to open the valves of your gallbladder so the fuel oil can move through and into your fire.

7. Rest for a moment. Then begin to pulse the mula bandha, or root lock. To do this, squeeze as if you were trying not to pee or poop. This is the oil pump, to get the oil moving and hold in the fire once we get the engine going. Squeeze the root lock back and forth fifteen times.

8. Next comes Breath of Fire, or kapalabati. Begin a series of quick exhalations, thrustings your breath out through your nose. Your belly will come back and your stomach muscles tighten during the exhalation. The inhalation will be a by-product of the exhalation, as the belly will naturally come back out. Now add in the liver mudra (triangle shape) as described above and the root lock, holding the root lock the whole time. Repeat fifteen times. This oxygen helps ignite the spark plugs and get the fire burning. If you feel sexually aroused, let that happen and add the energy to your fire focus spot. Rest.

9. Now do the same thing, but slow your breath. Breathing slowly as before, rock your hips back and forth and add the liver mudra and root lock. This time, however, do the root lock only on your inhalation as your abdomen and belly come forward. Continue this for fifteen repetitions.

10. Now that the belly fire is hot and burning and the engine is running, we are going to bring the fire up your spine. Imagine that each vertebra is like a tea candle and that the fire from your belly is going to light each candle all the way up to your head. Start to take a belly breath, squeezing the root lock and arching your back forward, and now focus on the fire coming up your spine to a point level with the kidneys, lighting each vertebra like a tea candle. Keep inhaling, bringing the breath all the way up from the belly into the chest and

as high up as you can. Let the breath move your body as you inhale. Your chest will expand at the peak of the inhalation, and your belly will flatten out some. Visualize or see the fire following the breath up your spine all the way to the center of your head. Imagine each tea candle being lit, one by one, as the fire goes up the vertebrae to the pineal and pituitary glands. Fill your body with as much breath as you can. Hold the root lock the whole time. This is the fire-up.

11. When you have filled your body with as much oxygen as you can, bring your chin down to your chest in a chin lock, and hold this lock and the root lock. Hold the breath and locks for as long as desired, in effect sealing your body with energy and oxygen. This is a good moment to set a prayer or intention for what it is you want. Exhale. Rest and go on to the next step when you are comfortable with these steps of the inhalation.

12. Repeat the inhalation, and now, with the locks in place and breath full, place the tip of your tongue at the roof of your mouth. This creates the channel for the fire energy that rises up to begin to come down the front of your body. Imagine the hot energy now being pulled down the front of your body. Let go of the root lock and begin to gently exhale out your mouth and around your tongue, which you hold in place as the energy comes down your tongue and into your chest. Smile.

13. Continue exhaling as the exhalation and energy now come down the front of your body. Imagine the hot fire that you brought up is now passing into your heart to be cooled in the radiator. Any negative thoughts can come down here from your mind as well. Allow a gentle sigh of release and relaxation to occur naturally.

14. Let the breath and exhalation continue down the front of your body into the solar plexus and intestines, carrying the love feeling generated from your heart. Imagine you are gently cradling the internal organs and belly as you continue to exhale with this blessed energy.

15. Allow for anything that has passed through your heart to now be digested in the fire in your belly. Feel the fire burn through and melt any impurities.

16. Let all the air come out and slump back a bit, naturally, as you finish the exhalation. Feel the energy loop back and cross over to your tailbone as you very gently push the root, as if you were going to the bathroom, and let any excess energy pass back into the earth to be recycled.

Go back to step 10 and repeat this cycle as often as you like. When you let your breath guide the movement, it ends up looking like a figure eight (from the side), so if it helps, you can imagine or emphasize the figure-eight movement as you follow the natural course of your breath.

This exercise is powerful and very healing as we use the power of fire and the energy of love to heal ourselves.

PART 2: LIBERATING WITH LOVE

After practicing and gaining competence with the Fire Love Generator described in part 1, you can now apply it to working with long-haul Covid or any other disease. Now are going to look at long Covid from a different angle, thanking it as our teacher, blessing it with all our love, and then, in part 3, liberating it with our fire.

1. After you have warmed up with the first part of the Fire Love Loop, picture Covid however you see it: as a spike protein or whatever works for you. Take this image and begin to feel how it is separate from you. Sense the differences. See how it might be similar, too. Also sense the connection and the interconnectedness that all life has. See it as a teacher: What's it trying to tell you? Come from a place of a nonjudgmental witness. Just watch as best you can. Is it possible to actually consider thanking it? Is it possible this disease is showing you where you have been out of balance?

2. Visualize a bright candle in the center of your heart. This is your love, your uniqueness, your spirit center, and the place of light that no one can ever take from you. Keep breathing and building this heart fire through your breath and the felt sense in the center of

your heart. Feel the things you love for a moment. Picture babies, people you love, trees, rivers, pets, Jesus—whatever it is you know you love. Imagine cradling your own heart as if it's the most sacred and beautiful thing in the world. Keep generating the feeling of unconditional love.

3. Once you have created love and are centered in your heart, take that image of Covid and love it with all your heart. To do this, either on the cool-down part of the Fire Love Generator or just with your heart, invite Covid in to be blessed. Invite it into your heart to get all the love you can give it. Take the image you have of Covid and hold it like a baby. Cradle it, kiss it, bless it, cherish it, rock it, and melt it in love. Use your hands to gently brush your body as well. No matter how disgusting, how vile, how scary Covid is, hold it. See it as part of the universe with a purpose. Keep returning to this again and again. Keep loving it with all your heart. Invite it in to be liberated or freed in the love of your heart. Picture it and feel it melting in your love. Rest in the idea that nothing can ever extinguish your heart fire.

The mind will rebel against this exercise, but keep returning again and again to this idea. This is a powerful and ancient exercise used by many monks, priests, holy ones, and avatars. Love heals. Love Covid again and again. Whenever you feel fear, frustration, anger, and hopelessness, stop and feel your heart. Think of what you love and pull the thoughts and Covid into the center of your heart to be blessed and transformed by love. When you do this exercise, you will find that Covid begins to lose power over you. How can something hurt you when you love it so much?

In my own experience in blessing the enemy, it took some time, but I kept returning to this exercise again and again. At a certain point I actually began to feel compassion for Covid. You can use this exercise for other "enemies," including thoughts and beliefs that are disempowering. Pull them into your heart to be transformed and then liberate them with our fire. Then it is much easier to pull out the "golden sword of transmutation" (see below, step 3). Always bless the enemy first as a part of creation. If it still wants to hurt you, you free it back to the universe, in a sense.

PART 3: LIBERATING WITH FIRE

This part of the exercise focuses on the hot fire coming up your spine and down to burn away disease. After practicing part 1 and blessing the enemy in part 2, you'll be ready to liberate Covid with fire.

1. Return to the feeling of hot fire in your belly. In the center of our planet is a hot molten ball of lava. In the core of our belly is a fiery molten core of lava that can transmute or melt anything back into its base. Imagine you are Frodo from *The Lord of the Rings* dropping the ring (Covid) from your heart back into the fire of your core to melt away.

2. Do part 1 (with fire breath, root lock, mudra, and spine rocking). Allow yourself to feel angry if it helps as a motivator. Set your intention. Imagine you are a tiger about to pounce on a gazelle. Do Breath of Fire thirty times.

3. When you're ready, hold the root lock, inhale, and bring the energy slowly up your spine (as in part 1). Pause and set your intention, and visualize yourself holding a golden sword of transmutation. On the exhale, open your mouth wide and breathe out like a dragon, as if you were breathing pure fire. Drop whatever is left of Covid into your belly fire. See all the hot fire you have generated burning and melting your image of Covid. Cut through it with your golden sword. (Another great image is picturing your belly like a giant composting digester and seeing whatever you have dropped in it being transmuted in this hot compost fire.)

4. Inhale through the nose again then exhale through your mouth, and imagine you are a dragon or tiger and growl, hiss, or gurgle (as if you were vomiting) on the exhale. Feel the sensation of embodying a warrior, burning anything in your way. You may feel like vomit-

ing, and so on the final part of the exhalation curl forward and feel how disgusting Covid makes you feel. Go through the motions of a vomit if needed and be sure to spit out what comes up.

This is where you liberate anything that wants to harm you. State your boundaries. Claim your body. Guard your temple. Light your fire. Stand firm against anything that would harm you. Stomp the ground. Roar. Go full on warrior-shaman. Use your sword. Push Covid off and out of you. Kick it in the ass. Burn it. Men, imagine or feel the energy of your testicles raging like a bull, and women, imagine the powerful energy of your ovaries transforming you into a lioness.

5. As before, at the end of the exhalation let any excess energy drain out your tailbone and back into the earth for composting.

6. Rest and see this fire you have generated pour into the red marrow in your bones, and see the immune system with all the white blood cells and other warrior cells come to eat and digest any Covid invaders.

7. Repeat part 2 of the exercise, and again bring the energy down into your heart to bless and love Covid.

8. As the energy comes back down into your belly, see whatever may be left melted in the hot lava core in the belly. Digest it. Break it back down.

9. Gently cool down by bringing your arms up over your head and down the sides of your body. Imagine a river of cooling water is washing through you from your crown to your tailbone.

APPENDIX 3

✦ ✦ ✦

Covid Panic
Emergency Meditation

IF YOU ARE HAVING a panic or anxiety attack:

1. Feel your feet. Place your awareness in your feet, and stay there as long as you can. Feel your legs: imagine you are a tree, firmly rooted.
2. Slow your breath, counting to four as you inhale, counting to six as you exhale while making a *shhh* sound. Create a mild tension in your stomach muscles if you can.
3. Close down your crown chakra. Imagine at the very top of your head a wheel of light spinning to the right and closing down. Keep it open just a crack, and only allow the highest light of the universe to come in.
4. Begin to think of the things you love: trees, mountains, pets, rivers, Mom, Dad, children, Jesus, Quan Yin, and so on. Generate the feeling of love. Hold it in your heart. What does that love feel like? Imagine a candle there in your heart, a flame that can never be extinguished.
5. Call on master angels (such as Michael) or Jesus or St. Germain or Mother Mary or whomever you trust in the spirit world to help you. Pour out love to them. Or call on a loved one who you trust.

6. Continue breathing deeply and slowly. Inhale and think *I am love.* Exhale and think or say *I love,* while thinking about love.

7. If you can, light a fire or a candle or gaze at the sun and begin to do Breath of Fire or the Fire Love Loop exercise (appendix 2) for twenty minutes while gazing into the flame. If you are not able to light a candle and you are lying in bed, breathe into your belly while holding a mild tension in your stomach muscles on both the inhalations and exhalations. Pulse the root lock (mula bandha) twenty times.

8. Drink some water. Lie back down and now imagine a cooling stream or river gently flowing through you, cleansing and calming your body.

9. Seal yourself with protection, such as the Violet Flame (see page 150), swords on all sides of you, horns on top of your head, armor, the seven mighty Elohim, Hercules, or whatever feels like protection.

10. Thank your guides, angels, and masters for helping.

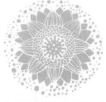

APPENDIX 4

✦ ✦ ✦

Healing Recipes, Tinctures, and Blends

THIS SECTION CONTAINS NOURISHING RECIPES for smoothies, drinks, soups, and tinctures that I've found especially useful. You'll need a good blender or Vitamix.

❀

Sodium Imbalance/Electrolyte/ Antihistamine Drink

½ teaspoon salt
½ teaspoon baking soda
Powdered vitamin C (3,000 mg)
Squeeze of lemon
Bit of honey

Stir all the ingredients into a glass of water and drink two or three times a day. I found this mix tremendously helpful.

· ·

Antihistamine Tea Options

- Boil 2 onions and 2 apples in a pot for 1 hour. Let cool and drink.
- Loose leaf herb teas: Panax ginseng, nettles, calendula, and/or chamomile

· ·

❀
Morning Smoothie

1 green apple or 2 scoops of apple pectin

1 lemon, with skin removed (beware any
    histamine reaction to the citrus)

2-inch piece of raw gingerroot

2-inch piece of raw turmeric root

1 avocado, peeled, but with its pit

Handful of blueberries and/or blackberries

Combine all the ingredients in sturdy blender and process until smooth.

❀
Raw Healing Soup

1 avocado, peeled, but with its pit

3 kale leaves

2 mustard green leaves

1 parsley sprig

1 cilantro sprig

1 lemon

2-inch piece of raw gingerroot

2-inch piece of raw turmeric root

1 teaspoon salt, or to taste

Pinch of dulse flakes

Pinch of ground cayenne

3 tablespoons olive oil

Combine all the ingredients in sturdy blender and process until smooth.

❁

Immune-Boosting Mushroom Milk

For the mushrooms, the powders of the fruiting bodies are best.

1 tablespoon chaga mushroom powder
1 tablespoon lion's mane mushroom powder
1 tablespoon reishi mushroom powder
1 tablespoon turkey tail mushroom powder
1 tablespoon colostrum powder
1 tablespoon ghee or raw cream
One small finger fresh turmeric
Pinch of ground cinnamon
Spoonful of honey
Raw milk or coconut milk to taste

Combine all the ingredients in sturdy blender and process until smooth.

❁

Colon Clearing Powder

Triphala is a powerful ayurvedic remedy consisting of three dried fruits native to India: bibhitaki, amalaki, and haritaki.

1 part ground psyllium seed
1 part triphala
1 part ground chia seed
1 part ground anise
1 part powdered clay (bentonite, food-grade)
1 part ground licorice root
½ part ground mustard seed
½ part ground ginger

Combine all the ingredients. Mix 1 to 2 tablespoons with grapefruit juice and drink first thing in the morning.

HERBAL TINCTURE BLENDS
FOR LONG COVID

The following are tincture blends I developed. To make your own tincture blends you can buy single tinctures and blend them or make your own tinctures. Consult an herbalist to do so. Typically the raw herb is extracted in alchohol or glycerin for a few weeks.

Use equal parts of each tincture for the following blends, except where indicated otherwise.

❀

Mold Drain Tincture

Dragon's blood

Ocotillo

Propolis

Nicotiana (use ⅓ part)

Take one dropperful two times a day, three times a week (every other day).

❀

Spike Soap Tincture

Fennel

Horse chestnut

Licorice

Agave (use ⅓ part)

Take one dropperful two times a day, three times a week (every other day). Alternate with Mold Drain Tincture.

❀
Brain Blend Tincture

American ginseng

Bacopa

Calendula

Ginkgo biloba

Gotu kola

Milky oats

Mint

Passionflower

Rosemary

Skullcap

Take two droppersful twice daily or as needed.

✦ ✦ ✦

Homeopathic Repertory for Covid Symptoms

Dosages: Try cycling through remedies one at a time to see what works for you. For acute situations take at 30C potency, three times a day, to halt the progression. For chronic conditions start with 200C two times the first day and then go to 30C three times a day. Try rotating or switching up remedies every five days, taking two or three times a day. Work with a homeopath for higher potencies (1M or more) for a more precise action.

ACUTE ONSET OF POSSIBLE COLD/COVID SYMPTOMS

- Aconite—for panic/fear/racing heart, restlessness, and coldness
- Arsenicum—for anxiety, restlessness, fear of exposure/germs, need for reassurance, burning skin
- Bryonia—wanting to be left alone, tiredness, irritability, need to veg out, forehead headache
- Gelsemium—for shakiness, anxiety, weakness, trembling

ACHES AND PAINS

- Arnica—for inability to get comfortable, feeling bruised, achiness, swelling, dislike of touch
- Baptisia—for feeling scattered, confused, sleepy, delirious, bruised, and uncomfortable
- Bryonia—for someone who wants to be left alone, tiredness, irritability, need to veg out, forehead headache
- Eupatorium—for pain that feels as if bones are broken, great thirst, back pain
- Gelsemium—for shakiness, anxiety, weakness, trembling
- Rhus toxicodendron—for achiness at first movement but improvement with more movement, restlessness, back pain, irritability, burning sensations

APATHY WITH BRAIN FOG

- Candida albicans—for feeling cloudy, spacey, itchy, giggling for no reason, history of yeast infections, symptoms worse with sugar consumption and damp weather
- Carboneum oxygenisatum—for coldness, sleepiness, loss of consciousness, vertigo, cerebral congestion
- Phosphoricum acidum—for feeling burnout, no energy left, flat emotions; needing naps and refreshing drinks. Other acid remedies such as Sulfuric acid and Picric acid may help with feelings of apathy as well.
- Virus nosodes such as Influenzinum and Oscillococcinum—for repetitive thoughts, insomnia, OCD-like behaviors

AUTOIMMUNITY
WITH JOINT INFLAMMATION

- Ignatia—for lump in the throat, suppressed grief and emotions, tremor, attacks of joint inflammation

- Lyme nosode remedies—if there is a history of Lyme exposure/infection and shifting joint pains.
- Rhus toxicodendron—for achiness of joints with first movement but improvement with more movement, restlessness, back pain, irritability; symptoms worse in damp weather
- Streptococcinum—for self-hate/self-attack, history of strep, sore throat, autoimmune conditions. Suppression of strep bacteria can predispose to autoimmune conditions.

BURNOUT AND FATIGUE

- Carboneum oxygenisatum—for coldness, sleepiness, loss of consciousness, vertigo, cerebral congestion
- Carbo vegetabilis—for weakness, gassiness, air hunger, depletion, coldness, cachectic states
- Carcinosinum—for suppressed immunity with lack of reaction (i.e., lack of fever response), often due to history of suppressive medication; insomnia; feelings of chaos, desire for control
- Epstein-Barr nosode—for exhaustion, need for a lot of sleep, history of EBV infection
- Nitricum acidum—for feeling irritable, peevish, cynical; herpes eruptions, cracks at corners of the mouth, warts; burned out on activity and adventure
- Phosphoricum acidum—for depression, apathy, indifference, especially if after loss/grief; craving of fresh juice and refreshing things; hair loss; burned out on relating to others
- Sulphuricum acidum—for feeling irritable, peevish, dissatisfied, hurried; cold sores, tendency to bruising; burned out on relationships and activity

CALMING THE LIMBIC SYSTEM/
AMYGDALA/BRAIN STEM

- Belladonna—for fight-or-flight response, dilated pupils, migraines, throbbing pains, sensory overwhelm

- Hyoscyamus—for relationship issues, jealousy, attachment, any/all kinds of pelvic/rectal/sexual issues
- Psychedelic remedies (Ayahuasca, Cannabis indica, Anhalonium, etc.)—for calming hallucinations and feeling "out of body"
- Reptile remedies (Lachesis, Crotalus horridus, etc.)—for calming the limbic system, especially if there is aggression, jealousy, and fear of constriction
- Stramonium—for nightmares, fear of death, fight-or-flight anxiety, sensory overwhelm

COUGH COMPLICATIONS

- Antimonium arsenicum—for cough with panting, breathlessness, acute respiratory distress, cyanosis
- Antimonium tartaricum—for cough accompanied by irritability, adverseness to being touch, weakened state, sleepiness during cough, cyanosis; cough is wet and rattling
- Carbo vegetabilis—for difficulty breathing when lying down, must sit up; desire for extra oxygen, to be fanned, or window opened, but feeling cold; fainting; coldness
- Justicia—for dry, spasmodic, constricted cough, threaten of suffocation, and tightness of chest, as if it would burst, with bronchial rattle
- Lobelia—for cough with panting, threat of suffocation, fear of death, dyspnea from constriction of chest that is worsened by any exertion, with sense of a lump in the stomach rising into the mouth and rattling in the chest but no expectoration
- Phosphorus—for tickling cough, made worse by talking, with oppression of chest and hoarseness
- Rumex crispus—for tickling in the throat, dry cough made worse from cold air or change in temperature; cough worse from pressure on the throat
- Spongia—for a hard dry cough, croupiness, with constricting and tickling in the throat

- Squilla—for a hard cough, either dry or loose, with loss of urine/stool during cough, and possibly with pneumonia

COVID TOES

- Agaricus muscarius—toes are as if frostbitten
- Petroleum—toes are dry, parched, with deep cracks in the skin

HAIR LOSS

- Ferrum phos—when anemia is the cause of hair loss
- Phosphoricum acidum—for apathy, burnout especially in relating to others, need for naps and fresh drinks
- Thuja—for insecure self-image, tendency to warts
- Thyroidinum—for thyroid support
- Ustilago—alopecia, itchy scalp, fungal involvement

HEADACHES/BRAIN INFLAMMATION

- Apis—for burning, swelling, itching, heat, crying out, symptoms that improve with cold
- Belladonna—for throbbing headache, occipital pain, symptoms that improve with low sensory input, sunburn
- Natrum muriaticum—for headache pain that is worse around eyes, worse in the morning upon waking, worse in the sun; for tendency toward overthinking, being introverted
- Nux vomica—for irritability, impatience, ambitiousness, craving for stimulants, symptoms that worsen with noise, light, or activity
- Stramonium—for nightmares, sensory sensitivity, primal fears arising with headaches

HEAVY DEPRESSION

- Aurum—for feeling great responsibility to others, pain around the heart, possible suicidal thoughts, symptoms that improve with music, spiritually inclined
- Bismuth—for very heavy feelings of depression, giving up, loneliness, suicidal thoughts; desires company and fears being alone; stomach pains
- Natrum muriaticum—for loneliness, being cut off from relationships, being sensitive to others but introverted
- Reptile remedies (like Dendroaspis or Lachesis)—for dark depression combined with jealousy and signs of heat/inflammation

LUNG STRENGTHENING

- Lung sarcode—to strengthen the function of the lungs
- Medhorrhinum—for adventurous people with history of asthma from childhood or chronic bronchitis, dyspnea; symptoms that improve when knees are brought to the chest
- Mycoplasma nosode—for a history of walking pneumonia, low-level depression
- Oxygenium—for victim mentality, feeling suffocated, history of low oxygenation at birth
- Phosphorus—for poor boundaries, excessive openness, friendliness, being made sad easily
- Pneumococcinum—if there is a history of bacterial pneumonia
- Stannum metallicum—for a hollow "tinny" cough with weakness, being too weak to talk
- Tuberculinum—for a desire to travel, cynicism, history of lung infection, history of smoking

MAST CELL ACTIVATION SYNDROME

- Agaricus—anxiety about health, twitches, spasms, for mold sensitivity as a histamine trigger
- Apis—for burning sensation, swelling around the eyes; symptom improvement with application of cold
- Belladonna—for heat, swelling, dilated pupils, migraines, fight-or-flight response
- Histaminum—take in low potency daily to reduce histamine levels
- Natrum muriaticum—for watery nasal discharge, hay fever, sadness with inability to weep

MENSTRUAL IRREGULARITIES AND PELVIC CONGESTION

- Aesculus—for varicose veins, hemorrhoids, venous stasis
- Bellis perennis—for feeling bruised around the pelvic area, for history of pelvic or birth trauma
- Hyoscyamus—for relationship issues, jealousy, attachment, need for attention, plus any/all kinds of pelvic/rectal/sexual issues
- Lachesis—for fullness, loquaciousness, heat; menopausal or perimenopausal
- Lilium tigrinum—for the feeling that pelvic organs will prolapse, PMS with great irritability; hypersexual
- Paeonia—hemorhhoids, strong attachment to mother, excitability and sensitivity, symptoms made worse by heat
- Pulsatilla—menstrual irregularity or shortness in duration, endometriosis
- Staphysagria—for indignation, need for attention, hypersensitivity, teariness

. . . .

Mental/Emotional Sphere

Fear of germs/excessive handwashing: Arsenicum, Syphilinum

Feeling of persecution: China officinalis, Cina, Oxygenium, Syphilinum

Feeling overwhelmed by chaos: Calcarea carbonica, Carcinosin

Negativity in general: Antimonium, Chlorum, Natrum muriaticum, Sepia, Tuberculinum

Sense of injustice: Causticum, Ignatia

Panic attacks: Aconitum, Adrenalinum, Arsenicum, Hyoscyamus niger, Rescue Remedy, Stramonium

Paranoia: Cannibis indica, Lachesis, Veratrum album

Cultural malaise/feeling dull, uninspired in the system, like the fun has been taken out of things, not wanting to leave home: Carboneum oxygenisatum, Graphites, Kali carbonicum, Natrum muriaticum

Feeling of isolation, social indifference, flat emotions: Lac humanum, Natrum muriaticum, Sepia

Addiction to devices (computers, cell phones, gaming devices, social media): Coffea cruda, Nux vomica, Thuja, Opium

Frustration and anger at the system: Anacardium, Causticum, China officinalis, Ignatia, Lachesis, Rhus toxicodendron

. . . .

SPIKE PROTEIN BREAKDOWN

- Petroleum—for chilliness, nausea, ravenous appetite, cracking of tissues, deep-seated stuck toxicity
- Graphites and Silica—for skin formation issues, issues with toenails, cracks in the skin, rashes, issues with pushing things out of the system
- Sulfuric acid—scattered mind and hurried; symptoms worse from exhaust and fumes; tendency to bruise
- Thuja—for a sense of inner fragility and a need to be tough on the outside; helps strengthen the inner sense of self

References

AAT Bioquest. 2020. How does alcohol denature a protein? AAT Bioquest website, June 22, 2020.

Abdelgawad, S. M., M. A. E. Hassab, M. A. S. Abourehab, E. B. Elkaeed, W. M. Eldehna. 2022. "Olive Leaves as a Potential Phytotherapy in the Treatment of COVID-19 Disease; a Mini-Review." *Frontiers in Pharmacology* 13. https://doi.org/10.3389/fphar.2022.879118.

Abdelmoaty, S., H. Arthur, I. Spyridopoulos, M. Wagberg, R. Fritsche Danielson, J. Pernow, A. Gabrielsen, and T. Olin. 2019. "5234. KAND567, the First Selective Small Molecule CX3CR1 Antagonist in Clinical Development, Mediates Anti-Inflammatory Cardioprotective Effects in Rodent Models of Atherosclerosis and Myocardial Infarction." *European Heart Journal* 40, no. 1: ehz746.0080. https://doi.org/10.1093/eurheartj/ehz746.0080.

Abubakar, Murtala Bello, Dawoud Usman, Gaber El-Saber Batiha, Natália Cruz-Martins, Ibrahim Malami, Kasimu Ghandi Ibrahim, Bilyaminu Abubakar, Muhammad Bashir Bello, Aliyu Muhammad, Siew Hua Gan et al. 2021. "Natural Products Modulating Angiotensin Converting Enzyme 2 (ACE2) as Potential COVID-19 Therapies." *Frontiers in Pharmacology* 12. https://doi.org/10.3389/fphar.2021.629935.

Achar, A., and C. Ghosh. 2020. "COVID-19-Associated Neurological Disorders: The Potential Route of CNS Invasion and Blood-Brain Relevance." *Cells* 9, no. 11: 2360. https://doi.org/10.3390/cells9112360.

Adusumilli, N. C., D. Zhang, J. M. Friedman, and A. J. Friedman. 2020. "Harnessing Nitric Oxide for Preventing, Limiting and Treating the Severe Pulmonary Consequences of Covid-19." *Nitric Oxide* 103: 4–8.

Ahmad, A., A. Husain, M. Mujeeb, et al. 2013. "A Review on Therapeutic Potential of Nigella sativa: A Miracle Herb." *Asian Pacific Journal of Tropical Biomedicine* 3, no. 5: 337–52. https://doi.org/10.1016/S2221-1691(13)60075-1.

Alam, S., S., Sadiqi, M. Sabir, S. Nisa, S. Ahmad, and S. W. Abbasi. 2022. "Bacillus Species; a Potential Source of Anti-SARS-CoV-2 Main Protease Inhibitors." *Journal of Biomolecular Structure and Dynamics* 40, no. 13: 5748–58. https://doi.org/10.1080/07391102.2021.1873188.

Alcaraz, M. J., and M. Payá. 2006. "Marine Sponge Metabolites for the Control of Inflammatory Diseases." *Current Opinion in Investigational Drugs* 7, no. 11: 974–79.

Alhazmi, H. A., A. Najmi, S. A. Javed, et al. 2021. "Medicinal Plants and Isolated Molecules Demonstrating Immunomodulation Activity as Potential Alternative Therapies for Viral Diseases Including COVID-19." *Frontiers in Immunology* 12: 637553. https://doi.org/10.3389/fimmu.2021.637553.

Ali, A., Y. Ma, J. Reynolds, J. P. Wise, S. E. Inzucchi, and D. L. Katz. 2011. "Chromium

Picolinate for the Prevention of Type 2 Diabetes." *Treatment Strategies: Diabetes* 3, no. 1: 34–40.

Ameya, G., A. Manilal, and B. Merdekios. 2017. "In Vitro Antibacterial Activity and Phytochemical Analysis of Nicotiana tabacum l. Extracted in Different Organic Solvents." *Open Microbiology Journal* 11: 352–59. https://doi.org/10.2174/1874285801711010352.

Andersson, M., M. Persson, and A. Kjellgren. 2017. "Psychoactive Substances as a Last Resort: A Qualitative Study of Self-Treatment of Migraine and Cluster Headaches." *Harm Reduction Journal* 14, no. 1: 60. https://doi.org/10.1186/s12954-017-0186-6.

Arenas, A., C. Borge, A. Carbonero, et al. 2021. "Bovine Coronavirus Immune Milk against COVID-19." *Frontiers in Immunology* 12: 637152. https://doi.org/10.3389/fimmu.2021.637152.

Arthur, John M., J. Craig Forrest, Karl W. Boehme, Joshua L. Kennedy, Shana Owens, Christian Herzog, Juan Liu, and Terry O. Harville. 2021. "Development of ACE2 Autoantibodies after SARS-CoV-2 Infection." *PLOS ONE* 16, no. 9: e0257016. https://doi.org/10.1371/journal.pone.0257016.

Asif, M., M. Saleem, M. Saadullah, H. S. Yaseen, and R. Al Zarzour. 2020. "COVID-19 and Therapy with Essential Oils Having Antiviral, Anti-inflammatory, and Immunomodulatory Properties." *Inflammopharmacology* 28, no. 5: 1153–61. https://doi.org/10.1007/s10787-020-00744-0.

Avolio, Elisa, Michele Carrabba, Rachel Milligan, Maia Kavanagh Williamson, Antonio P. Beltrami, Kapil Gupta, Karen T. Elvers et al. 2021. "The SARS-CoV-2 Spike Protein Disrupts Human Cardiac Pericytes Function through CD147 Receptor-Mediated Signalling: A Potential Non-infective Mechanism of COVID-19 Microvascular Disease." *Clinical Science (London)* 135, no. 24: 2667–89. https://doi.org/10.1042/CS20210735.

Ayoobi, F., A. Shamsizadeh, I. Fatemi, A. Vakilian, M. Allahtavakoli, G. Hassanshahi, and A. Moghadam-Ahmadi. 2017. "Bio-effectiveness of the Main Flavonoids of *Achillea millefolium* in the Pathophysiology of Neurodegenerative Disorders—a Review." *Iranian Journal of Basic Medical Sciences* 20, no. 6: 604–12. https://doi.org/10.22038/IJBMS.2017.8827.

Ayoubkhani, D., C. Bermingham, K. B. Pouwels, M. Glickman, V. Nafilyan, F. Zaccardi, et al. 2022. "Trajectory of Long Covid Symptoms after Covid-19 Vaccination: Community Based Cohort Study." 377. https://doi.org/10.1136/bmj-2021-069676.

Baba, M., O. Nishimura, N. Kanzaki, et al. 1999. "A Small-Molecule, Nonpeptide CCR5 Antagonist with Highly Potent and Selective Anti-HIV-1 Activity." *Proceedings of the National Academy of Sciences of the United States of America* 96, no. 10: 5698–703. https://doi.org/10.1073/pnas.96.10.5698.

Barletta, M. A., G. Marino, B. Spagnolo, et al. 2022. "Coenzyme Q10 + Alpha Lipoic Acid for Chronic COVID Syndrome. *Clinical and Experimental Medicine*. https://doi.org/10.1007/s10238-022-00871-8

Barré, J., J.-M. Sabatier, and C. Annweiler. 2020. "Montelukast Drug May Improve COVID-19 Prognosis: A Review of Evidence." *Frontiers in Pharmacology* 11: 1344. https://doi.org/10.3389/fphar.2020.01344.

Barrett, C. E., A. K. Koyama, P. Alvarez, et al. 2022. "Risk for Newly Diagnosed Diabetes > 30 Days after SARS-CoV-2 Infection among Persons Aged < 18 Years—United States, March 1, 2020–June 28, 2021." *Morbidity and Mortality Weekly Report* 71: 59–65. https://doi.org/10.15585/mmwr.mm7102e2external icon.

Barroso-González, J., N. El Jaber-Vazdekis, L. García-Expósito, et al. 2009. "The Lupane-Type Triterpene 30-Oxo-Calenduladiol Is a CCR5 Antagonist with Anti-HIV-1 and Anti-chemotactic Activities." *Journal of Biological Chemistry* 284, no. 24: 16609–20. https://doi.org/10.1074/jbc.M109.005835.

Basil, M. C., and B. D. Levy. 2016. "Specialized Pro-resolving Mediators: Endogenous Regulators of Infection and Inflammation." *Natural Reviews Immunology* 16, no. 1: 51–67. https://doi.org/10.1038/nri.2015.4.

Bennett, Doug. 2020. "Existing Antihistamine Drugs Show Effectiveness against COVID-19 Virus in Cell Testing." UFHealth (online), December 3, 2020.

Bent, S., A. Padula, D. Moore, M. Patterson, and W. Mehling. 2006. "Valerian for Sleep: A Systematic Review and Meta-analysis." *American Journal of Medicine* 119, no. 12: 1005–12. https://doi.org/10.1016/j.amjmed.2006.02.026.

Berretta, Andresa Aparecida, Marcelo Augusto Duarte Silveira, José Manuel Cóndor Capcha, and David De Jong. 2020. "Propolis and Its Potential against SARS-CoV-2 Infection Mechanisms and COVID-19 Disease: Running Title: Propolis against SARS-CoV-2 Infection and COVID-19." *Biomedicine & Pharmacotherapy* 131: 110622.

Besedovsky, L., T. Lange, and J. Born. 2012. "Sleep and Immune Function." *Pflügers Archiv: European Journal of Physiology* 463, no. 1: 121–37.

Beshay, S., J. G. Youssef, F. Zahiruddin, M. Al-Saadi, S. Yau, A. Goodarzi, H. Huang, and J. Javitt. 2021. "Rapid Clinical Recovery from Critical COVID-19 Pneumonia with Vasoactive Intestinal Peptide Treatment. *Journal of Heart and Lung Transplantation* 40, no. 4. https://doi.org/10.1016/j.healun.2021.01.2036.

Bhattacharyya, D. 2020. "Reposition of Montelukast Either Alone or in Combination with Levocetirizine against SARS-CoV-2." *Medical Hypotheses* 144: 110046. https://doi.org/10.1016/j.mehy.2020.110046.

Bizzarri, M., A. S. Laganà, D. Aragona, and V. Unfer. 2020. "Inositol and Pulmonary Function. Could Myo-inositol Treatment Downregulate Inflammation and Cytokine Release Syndrome in SARS-CoV-2?" *European Review for Medical and Pharmacological Sciences* 24, no. 6: 3426–32. https://doi.org/10.26355/eurrev_202003_20715.

Blum, Vinicius Fontanesi, Sérgio Cimerman, James R. Hunter, Paulo Tierno, Acioly Lacerda, Alexandre Soeiro, et al. 2021. "Nitazoxanide Superiority to Placebo to Treat Moderate COVID-19: A Pilot Prove of Concept Randomized Double-Blind Clinical Trial." *eClinicalMedicine* 37: 100981

Bochkov, D. V., S. V. Sysolyatin, A. I. Kalashnikov, and I. A. Surmacheva. 2012. "Shikimic Acid: Review of Its Analytical, Isolation, and Purification Techniques from Plant and Microbial Sources." *Journal of Chemical Biology* 5, no. 1: 5–17. https://doi.org/10.1007/s12154-011-0064-8.

Boglione, L., G. Meli, F. Poletti, R. Rostagno, R. Moglia, M. Cantone, M. Esposito, C. Scianguetta, B. Domenicale, F. Di Pasquale, and S. Borrè. 2022. "Risk Factors and Incidence of Long-COVID Syndrome in Hospitalized Patients: Does Remdesivir Have a Protective Effect?" *QJM: An International Journal of Medicine* 114, no. 12: 865–71.

Boldrini, M., P. D. Canoll, and R. S. Klein. 2021. "How COVID-19 Affects the Brain." *JAMA Psychiatry* 78, no. 6: 682–83. https://doi.org/10.1001/jamapsychiatry.2021.0500.

Bolton, M. J., B. P. Chapman, and H. Van Marwijk. 2020. "Low-Dose Naltrexone as a Treatment for Chronic Fatigue Syndrome." *BMJ Case Reports* 13: e232502.

Bordes, S. J., S. Phang-Lyn, E. Najera, et al. 2021. "Pituitary Apoplexy Attributed to COVID-19 Infection in the Absence of an Underlying Macroadenoma or Other Identifiable Cause." *Cureus* 13, no. 2: e13315. https://doi.org/10.7759/cureus.13315.

Bostancıklıoğlu, M. 2020. "SARS-CoV2 Entry and Spread in the Lymphatic Drainage System of the Brain." *Brain, Behavior, and Immunity* 87: 122–23. https://doi.org/10.1016/j.bbi.2020.04.080.

Bozkurt, H. S., and E. M. Quigley. 2020. "The Probiotic Bifidobacterium in the Management of Coronavirus: A Theoretical Basis." *International Journal of Immunopathology and Pharmacology* 34: 2058738420961304. https://doi.org/10.1177/2058738420961304.

Breit, Sigrid, Aleksandra Kupferberg, Gerhard Rogler, and Gregor Hasler. 2018. "Vagus Nerve as Modulator of the Brain–Gut Axis in Psychiatric and Inflammatory Disorders." *Frontiers in Psychiatry* 9: 44.

Brown, D. P., D. T. Rogers, F. Pomerleau, K. B. Siripurapu, M. Kulshrestha, G. A. Gerhardt, and J. M. Littleton. 2016. "Novel Multifunctional Pharmacology of Lobinaline, the Major Alkaloid from Lobelia cardinalis." *Fitoterapia* 111: 109–23. https://doi.org/10.1016/j.fitote.2016.04.013.

Bryant, Andrew, Theresa A. Lawrie, Therese Dowswell, Edmund J. Fordham, Scott Mitchell, Sarah R. Hill, and Tony C. Tham. 2021. "Ivermectin for Prevention and Treatment of COVID-19 Infection: A Systematic Review, Meta-analysis, and Trial Sequential Analysis to Inform Clinical Guidelines." *American Journal of Therapeutics* 28, no. 4: e434-e460. https://doi.org/10.1097/MJT.0000000000001402.

Buonsenso, D., D. Munblit, C. De Rose, D. Sinatti, A. Ricchiuto, A. Carfi, and P. Valentini. 2021. "Preliminary Evidence on Long COVID in Children. *Acta Paediatrica* 110, no. 7: 2208–11. https://doi.org/10.1111/apa.15870.

Burchill, E., E. Lymberopoulos, E. Menozzi, S. Budhdeo, J. R. McIlroy, J. Macnaughtan, and N. Sharma. 2021. "The Unique Impact of COVID-19 on Human Gut Microbiome Research." *Frontiers in Medicine* 8: 652464. https://doi.org/10.3389/fmed.2021.652464.

Campbell-McBride, D. N. 2004. *Gut and Psychology Syndrome.* Cambridge, U.K.: Mediform.

Carabotti, M., A. Scirocco, M. A. Maselli, and C. Severi. 2015. "The Gut-Brain Axis: Interactions between Enteric Microbiota, Central and Enteric Nervous Systems." *Annals of Gastroenterology* 28, no. 2: 203–9.

Carlsen, M. H., B. L. Halvorsen, K. Holte, et al. 2010. "The Total Antioxidant Content of More Than 3100 Foods, Beverages, Spices, Herbs and Supplements Used Worldwide." *Nutrition Journal* 29: 3. https://doi.org/10.1186/1475-2891-9-3.

Caruso, A. A., A. Del Prete, A. I. Lazzarino, R. Capaldi, and L. Grumetto. 2020. "Might Hydrogen Peroxide Reduce the Hospitalization Rate and Complications of SARS-CoV-2 Infection?" *Infection Control & Hospital Epidemiology* 41, no. 11: 1360–61. https://doi.org/10.1017/ice.2020.170.

Castaño, G., R. Mas, L. Fernández, J. Illnait, R. Gámez, and E. Alvarez. 2001. "Effects of Policosanol 20 versus 40 mg/day in the Treatment of Patients with Type II Hypercholesterolemia: A 6-Month Double-Blind Study." *International Journal of Clinical Pharmacology Research* 21, no. 1: 43–57.

Cattel, F., S. Giordano, C. Bertiond, et al. 2021. "Ozone Therapy in COVID-19: A Narrative Review." *Virus Research* 291: 198207. https://doi.org/10.1016/j.virusres.2020.198207.

Centers for Disease Control and Prevention (CDC). Long Covid Household Pulse Survey 2022. https://www.cdc.gov/nchs/covid19/pulse/long-covid.htm

Cervia, C., Y. Zurbuchen, P. Taeschler, et al. 2022. "Immunoglobulin Signature Predicts Risk of Post-Acute COVID-19 Syndrome." *Nature Communications* 13: 446. https://doi.org/10.1038/s41467-021-27797-1

Chai, S. C., K. Davis, Z. Zhang, L. Zha, and K. F. Kirschner. 2019. "Effects of Tart Cherry Juice on Biomarkers of Inflammation and Oxidative Stress in Older Adults." *Nutrients* 11, no. 2: 228. https://doi.org/10.3390/nu11020228.

Chang, C. H., W. C. Tsai, M. S. Lin, Y. H. Hsu, and J. H. Pang. 2011. "The Promoting

Effect of Pentadecapeptide BPC 157 on Tendon Healing Involves Tendon Outgrowth, Cell Survival, and Cell Migration." *Journal of Applied Physiology* 110, no. 3: 774–80. https://doi.org/10.1152/japplphysiol.00945.2010.

Chatterjee, P., M. Ponnapati, C. Kramme, et al. 2020. "Targeted Intracellular Degradation of SARS-CoV-2 via Computationally Optimized Peptide Fusions." *Communications Biology* 3: 715. https://doi.org/10.1038/s42003-020-01470-7.

Chee, P. Y., M. Mang, E. S. Lau, et al. 2019. "Epinecidin-1, an Antimicrobial Peptide Derived from Grouper (Epinephelus coioides): Pharmacological Activities and Applications." *Frontiers in Microbiology* 10: 2631. https://doi.org/10.3389/fmicb.2019.02631.

Chen, J., and L. Vitetta. 2021. "Modulation of Gut Microbiota for the Prevention and Treatment of COVID-19." *Journal of Clinical Medicine* 10, no. 13: 2903. https://doi.org/10.3390/jcm10132903.

Chen, X., L. Yang, N. Zhang, et al. 2003. "Shikonin, a Component of Chinese Herbal Medicine, Inhibits Chemokine Receptor Function and Suppresses Human Immunodeficiency Virus Type 1." *Antimicrobial Agents and Chemotherapy* 47, no. 9: 2810–16. https://doi.org/10.1128/AAC.47.9.2810-2816.2003.

Chen, Y., Y. N. Zhang, R. Yan, et al. 2021. "ACE2-Targeting Monoclonal Antibody as Potent and Broad-Spectrum Coronavirus Blocker." *Signal Transduction and Targeted Therapy* 6: 315. https://doi.org/10.1038/s41392-021-00740-y.

Chertow, Daniel, Sydney Stein, Sabrina Ramelli, et al. 2021. "SARS-CoV-2 Infection and Persistence throughout the Human Body and Brain." Research Square preprint (version 1). https://doi.org/10.21203/rs.3.rs-1139035/v1.

Chevalier, G., S. T. Sinatra, J. L. Oschman, K. Sokal, and P. Sokal. 2012. "Earthing: Health Implications of Reconnecting the Human Body to the Earth's Surface Electrons. *Journal of Environmental and Public Health* 2012: 291541. https://doi.org/10.1155/2012/291541.

Choi, S. Y., and K. Park. 2016. "Effect of Inhalation of Aromatherapy Oil on Patients with Perennial Allergic Rhinitis: A Randomized Controlled Trial." *Evidence-Based Complementary and Alternative Medicine* 2016: 7896081. https://doi.org / 10.1155/2016/7896081.

Choudhury, A., N. C. Das, R. Patra, M. Bhattacharya, P. Ghosh, B. C. Patra, and S. Mukherjee. 2021. "Exploring the Binding Efficacy of Ivermectin against the Key Proteins of SARS-CoV-2 Pathogenesis: An In Silico Approach." *Future Virology* 16, no. 4. https://doi.org/10.2217/fvl-2020-0342.

Clark, H. 1995. *The Cure for All Diseases*. Chula Vista, Calif.: New Century Press.

———. 2004. *The Prevention of All Cancers*. Chula Vista, Calif.: New Century Press.

Colunga Biancatelli, R. M. L., P. A. Solopov, E. R. Sharlow, J. S. Lazo, P. E. Marik, and J. D. Catravas. 2021. "The SARS-CoV-2 Spike Protein Subunit S1 Induces COVID-19-like Acute Lung Injury in K18-hACE2 Transgenic Mice and Barrier Dysfunction in Human Endothelial Cells." *American Journal of Physiology: Lung Cellular and Molecular Physiology* 321, no. 2: L477–84. https://doi.org/10.1152/ajplung.00223.2021.

Conti, P., A. Caraffa, G. Tetè, C. E. Gallenga, R. Ross, S. K. Kritas, I. Frydas, A. Younes, P. Di Emidio, and G. Ronconi. 2020. "Mast Cells Activated by SARS-CoV-2 Release Histamine Which Increases IL-1 levels Causing Cytokine Storm and Inflammatory Reaction in COVID-19." *Journal of Biological Regulators and Homeostatic Agents* 34, no. 5: 1629–32. https://doi.org/10.23812/20-2EDIT.

Cory, T. J., R. S. Emmons, J. R. Yarbro, et al. 2021. "Metformin Suppresses Monocyte Immunometabolic Activation by SARS-CoV-2 and Spike Protein Subunit 1." *Frontiers in Immunology*. https://doi.org/10.3389/fimmu.2021.733921.

Costa, L. H. A., B. M. Santos, and L. G. S. Branco. 2020. "Can Selective Serotonin Reuptake Inhibitors Have a Neuroprotective Effect during COVID-19?" *European Journal of Pharmacology* 889: 173629. https://doi.org/10.1016/j.ejphar.2020.173629.

COVID-19 Early Treatment Fund (CETF). 2022. Fluvoxamine data for COVID-19 Treatment. COVID-19 Early Treatment Fund website.

Cross, M. L., and H. S. Gill. 2000. "Immunomodulatory Properties of Milk." *British Journal of Nutrition* 84, suppl. 1: S81–89. https://doi.org/10.1017/s0007114500002294.

Cuadrado, Antonio, Marta Pajares, Cristina Benito, José Jiménez-Villegas, Maribel Escoll, Raquel Fernández-Ginés, Angel J. Garcia Yagüe, Diego Lastra, Gina Manda, Ana I. Rojo, and Albena T. Dinkova-Kostova. 2020. "Can Activation of NRF2 Be a Strategy against COVID-19?" *Trends in Pharmacological Sciences* 41, no. 9. https://doi.org/10.1016/j.tips.2020.07.003.

Dani, Melanie, Andreas Dirksen, Patricia Taraborrelli, Miriam Torocastro, Dimitrios Panagopoulos, Richard Sutton, and Phang Boon Lim. 2021. "Autonomic Dysfunction in 'Long COVID': Rationale, Physiology and Management Strategies." *Clinical Medicine Journal* 21, no. 1: e63–67. https://doi.org/10.7861/clinmed.2020-0896.

Dağ, Ş., H. Özpınar, M. Sarı, and N. Özpınar. 2015. "Antimicrobial Effect of Cola on Several Microorganisms." *Cumhuriyet Üniversitesi Fen Edebiyat Fakültesi Fen Bilimleri Dergisi* 36, no. 1: 52–59.

Decaux, G., F. Gankam Kengne, B. Couturier, F. Vandergheynst, W. Musch, and A. Soupart. 2014. "Actual Therapeutic Indication of an Old Drug: Urea for Treatment of Severely Symptomatic and Mild Chronic Hyponatremia Related to SIADH." *Journal of Clinical Medicine* 3, no. 3: 1043–49. https://doi.org/10.3390/jcm3031043.

del Valle-Mendoza, J., Y. Tarazona-Castro, A. Merino-Luna, et al. 2022. "Comparison of Cytokines Levels among COVID-19 Patients Living at Sea Level and High Altitude." *BMC Infectious Diseases* 22: 96. https://doi.org/10.1186/s12879-022-07079-x.

de Vos, Cato M. H., Natasha L. Mason, and Kim P. C. Kuypers. 2021. "Psychedelics and Neuroplasticity: A Systematic Review Unraveling the Biological Underpinnings of Psychedelics." *Frontiers in Psychiatry* 12: 724606. https://doi.org/10.3389/fpsyt.2021.724606.

Dilokthornsakul, W., R. Kosiyaporn, R. Wuttipongwaragon, P. Dilokthornsakul. 2022. "Potential Effects of Propolis and Honey in COVID-19 Prevention and Treatment: A Systematic Review of in Silico and Clinical Studies." *Journal of Integrative Medicine* 20, no. 2: 114–25. https://doi.org/10.1016/j.joim.2022.01.008.

Distinguin, L., A. Ammar, J. R. Lechien, et al. 2021. "MRI of Patients Infected with COVID-19 Revealed Cervical Lymphadenopathy." *Ear, Nose & Throat Journal* 100, no. 1: 26–28. https://doi.org/10.1177/0145561320940117.

Douaud, G., S. Lee, F. Alfaro-Almagro, et al. 2022. "SARS-CoV-2 Is Associated with Changes in Brain Structure in UK Biobank." *Nature* 604: 697–707. https://doi.org/10.1038/s41586-022-04569-5.

Dudek-Makuch, Marlena, and Elżbieta Studzińska-Sroka. 2015. "Horse Chestnut— Efficacy and Safety in Chronic Venous Insufficiency: An Overview." *Revista Brasileira de Farmacognosia* 25, no. 5: 533–41.

Dufour, I., A. Werion, L. Belkhir, et al. 2021. "Serum Uric Acid, Disease Severity and Outcomes in COVID-19." *Critical Care* 25: 212. https://doi.org/10.1186/s13054-021-03616-3.

Eberle, R. J., D. S. Olivier, M. S. Amaral, I. Gering, D. Willbold, R. K. Arni, and M. A. Coronado. 2021. "The Repurposed Drugs Suramin and Quinacrine Cooperatively Inhibit SARS-CoV-2 3CL^{pro} In Vitro." *Viruses* 13, no. 5: 873. https://doi.org/10.3390/v13050873.

Ejelonu, Oluwamodupe Cecilia, Olusola Olalekan Elekofehinti, and Isaac Gbadura Adanlawo. 2017. "Tithonia diversifolia Saponin-Blood Lipid Interaction and

Its Influence on Immune System of Normal Wistar Rats." *Biomedicine & Pharmacotherapy* 87: 589–95. https://doi.org/10.1016/j.biopha.2017.01.017.

Ellingson, D-M., S. Kelner, G. Loseth, J. Wessberg, and H. Olausson. 2015. "The Neurology Shaping Affective Touch: Expectation, Motivation, and Meaning in the Multisensory Context," *Frontiers in Psychology* (January 6).

Emoto, M. 2001. *The Hidden Messages in Water.* Translated by D. A. Thayne. Hillsboro, Oreg.: Beyond Words.

Eroğlu, İ., B. Ç. Eroğlu, and G. S. Güven. 2021. "Altered Tryptophan Absorption and Metabolism Could Underlie Long-Term Symptoms in Survivors of Coronavirus Disease 2019 (COVID-19)." *Nutrition* 90: 111308. https://doi.org/10.1016/j.nut.2021.111308.

Escobar-Sánchez, M. L., L. Sánchez-Sánchez, and J. Sandoval-Ramírez. 2015. "Steroidal Saponins and Cell Death in Cancer." In *Cell Death: Autophagy, Apoptosis and Necrosis,* edited by Tobias Ntuli. London: IntechOpen. https://doi.org/10.5772/61438.

Farhadi, S. A., E. Bracho-Sanchez, S. L. Freeman, B. G. Keselowsky, and G. A. Hudalla. 2018. "Enzymes as Immunotherapeutics." *Bioconjugate Chemistry* 29, no. 3: 64956. https://doi.org/10.1021/acs.bioconjchem.7b00719.

Feder, Adriana, Sarah B. Rutter, Daniela Schiller, and Dennis S. Charney. 2020. "The Emergence of Ketamine as a Novel Treatment for Posttraumatic Stress Disorder." *Advances in Pharmacology* 89: 261–86.

Flanagan, Thomas W., and Charles D. Nichols. 2018. "Psychedelics as Antiinflammatory Agents." *International Review of Psychiatry* 30, no. 4: 363–75. https://doi.org/10.10 80/09540261.2018.1481827.

Fogarty, Helen, Liam Townsend, Hannah Morrin, Azaz Ahmad, Claire Comerford, Ellie Karampini, Hanna Englert, et al. 2021. "Persistent Endotheliopathy in the Pathogenesis of Long COVID Syndrome." *Journal of Thrombosis and Haemostasis* 19, no. 10. https://doi.org/10.1111/jth.15490.

Fox, Glenn. 2017. "What Science Reveals about Gratitude's Impact on the Brain." *Greater Good Magazine* (online), August 4, 2017.

Frara, S, A. Allora, L. Castellino, L. di Filippo, P. Loli, and A. Giustina. 2021. "COVID-19 and the Pituitary." *Pituitary* 24, no. 3:465–81. https://doi.org/10.1007 /s11102-021-01148-1.

Fritsche, K. L. 2015. "The Science of Fatty Acids and Inflammation." *Advances in Nutrition* 6, no. 3: 293S–301S. https://doi.org/10.3945/an.114.006940.

Front Line COVID-19 Critical Care Alliance (FLCCC). 2022. "I Recover: Post-Vaccine Treatment Protocol." FLCCC website, updated January 29, 2022.

Fuglsang, C. H., T. Johansen, K. Kaila, H. Kasch, and F. W. Bach. 2018. "Treatment of Acute Migraine by a Partial Rebreathing Device: A Randomized Controlled Pilot Study." *Cephalalgia* 38, no. 10: 1632–43. https://doi.org/10.1177/0333102418797285.

Ganji, Riya, and P. H. Reddy. 2021. "Impact of COVID-19 on Mitochondrial-Based Immunity in Aging and Age-Related Diseases." *Frontiers in Aging Neuroscience* 12: 614650. https://doi.org/10.3389/fnagi.2020.614650.

Garcia-Gutierrez, E., A. Narbad, and J. M. Rodríguez. 2020. "Autism Spectrum Disorder Associated with Gut Microbiota at Immune, Metabolomic, and Neuroactive Level." *Frontiers in Neuroscience* 14: 578666. https://doi.org/10.3389/fnins.2020.578666.

Gates, D. A. 2011. *The Body Ecology Diet: Regaining Your Health and Recovering Your Immunity.* New York: Hay House.

Geier, M. R., and D. A. Geier. 2020. "Respiratory Conditions in Coronavirus Disease 2019 (COVID-19): Important Considerations Regarding Novel Treatment Strategies to Reduce Mortality." *Medical Hypotheses* 140: 109760. https://doi.org/10.1016 /j.mehy.2020.109760.

Geraghty, K., M. Hann, and S. Kurtev. 2019. "Myalgic Encephalomyelitis/Chronic Fatigue Syndrome Patients' Reports of Symptom Changes Following Cognitive Behavioural Therapy, Graded Exercise Therapy and Pacing Treatments: Analysis of a Primary Survey Compared with Secondary Surveys." *Journal of Health Psychology* 24, no. 10: 1318–33. https://doi.org/10.1177/1359105317726152.

Gerson, C. 2007. *Healing the Gerson Way: Healing Cancer and Other Chronic Diseases.* Del Mar, Calif.: Totality Books.

Ghahestani, S. M., E. Shahab, S. Karimi, and M. H. Madani. 2020. "Methylene Blue May Have a Role in the Treatment of COVID-19." *Medical Hypotheses* 144. https://doi.org/10.1016/j.mehy.2020.110163.

Giam, Xingli. 2017. "Global Biodiversity Loss from Tropical Deforestation." *Proceedings of the National Academy of Sciences of the United States of America* 114, no. 23: 5775–77. https://doi.org/10.1073/pnas.1706264114.

Gioia, M., C. Ciaccio, P. Calligari, et al. 2020. "Role of Proteolytic Enzymes in the COVID-19 Infection and Promising Therapeutic Approaches." *Biochemical Pharmacology* 182: 114225. https://doi.org/10.1016/j.bcp.2020.114225.

Giri, R. K., V. Rajagopal, and V. K. Kalra. 2004. "Curcumin, the Active Constituent of Turmeric, Inhibits Amyloid Peptide-Induced Cytochemokine Gene Expression and CCR5-Mediated Chemotaxis of THP-1 Monocytes by Modulating Early Growth Response-1 Transcription Factor." *Journal of Neurochemistry* 91, no. 5: 1199–210. https://doi.org/10.1111/j.1471-4159.2004.02800.x.

Gold, J. E., R. A. Okyay, W. E. Licht, and D. J. Hurley. 2021. "Investigation of Long COVID Prevalence and Its Relationship to Epstein-Barr Virus Reactivation. Pathogens." *Pathogens* 10, no. 6: 763. https://doi.org/10.3390/pathogens10060763.

Gonzalez, J. G., G. delle Monache, F. delle Monache, and G. B. Marini-Bettolò. 1982. "Chuchuhuasha—a Drug Used in Folk Medicine in the Amazonian and Andean Areas. A Chemical Study of Maytenus laevis." *Journal of Ethnopharmacology* 5, no. 1: 73–77. https://doi.org/10.1016/0378-8741(82)90022-8.

Groff, D., A. Sun, A. E. Ssentongo, et al. 2021. "Short-Term and Long-Term Rates of Postacute Sequelae of SARS-CoV-2 Infection: A Systematic Review." *JAMA Network Open* 4, no. 10: e2128568. https://doi.org/10.1001/jamanetworkopen.2021.28568.

Guggenheim, A. G., K. M. Wright, and H. L. Zwickey. 2014. "Immune Modulation from Five Major Mushrooms: Application to Integrative Oncology." *Integrative Medicine* 13, no. 1: 32–44.

Guilliams, T. G., and L. E. Drake. 2020. "Meal-Time Supplementation with Betaine HCL for Functional Hypochlorhydria: What Is the Evidence?" *Integrative Medicine* (Encinitas) 19, no. 1: 32–36.

Gupta, A., Y. Gonzalez-Rojas, E. Juarez, et al. 2021. "Early Treatment for Covid-19 with SARS-CoV-2 Neutralizing Antibody Sotrovimab." *New England Journal of Medicine* 385, no. 21: 1941–50.

Hagen, C., M. Nowack, M. Messerli, F. Saro, F. Mangold, and P. K. Bode. 2021. "Fine Needle Aspiration in COVID-19 Vaccine-Associated Lymphadenopathy." *Swiss Medical Weekly* 151: w20557. https://doi.org/10.4414/smw.2021.20557.

Hall, S. S. 2011. "Unfrozen." *National Geographic,* November 1, 2011.

Hamed, M. G. M., and R. S. Hagag. 2020. "The Possible Immunoregulatory and Anti-inflammatory Effects of Selective Serotonin Reuptake Inhibitors in Coronavirus Disease Patients." *Medical Hypotheses* 144: 110140. https://doi.org/10.1016/j.mehy.2020.110140.

Hannan, M. A., M. A. Rahman, M. S. Rahman, et al. 2020. "Intermittent Fasting, a Possible Priming Tool for Host Defense against Sars-Cov-2 Infection: Crosstalk among Calorie Restriction, Autophagy and Immune Response." *Immunology Letters* 226: 38-45. https://doi.org/10.1016/j.imlet.2020.07.001.

Hatanaka, N., B. Xu, M. Yasugi, H. Morino, H. Tagishi, T. Miura, T. Shibata, and S. Yamasaki. 2021. "Chlorine Dioxide Is a More Potent Antiviral Agent against Sars-Cov-2 Than Sodium Hypochlorite." *Journal of Hospital Infection* 118: 20-26.

Heinz, F. X., and K. Stiasny. 2021. "Distinguishing Features of Current COVID-19 Vaccines: Knowns and Unknowns of Antigen Presentation and Modes of Action." *npj Vaccines* 6, no. 104. https://doi.org/10.1038/s41541-021-00369-6.

Helfer, M., H. Koppensteiner, M. Schneider, S. Rebensburg, S. Forcisi, et al. 2014. "The Root Extract of the Medicinal Plant Pelargonium sidoides Is a Potent HIV-1 Attachment Inhibitor." *PLOS ONE* 9, no. 1: e87487. https://doi.org/10.1371/journal.pone.0087487.

Helsingin yliopisto (University of Helsinki). 2015. "Listening to Classical Music Modulates Genes That Are Responsible for Brain Functions." ScienceDaily (webpage).

Herrera-Ruiz, M., E. Jiménez-Ferrer, J. Tortoriello, et al. 2021. "Anti-neuroinflammatory Effect of Agaves and Cantalasaponin-1 in a Model of LPS-Induced Damage. *Natural Product Research* 35, no. 5: 884-87. https://doi.org/10.1080/14786419.2019.1608537.

Hesselink, Jan M. Keppel. 2018. "Kambo: A Ritualistic Healing Substance from an Amazonian Frog and a Source of New Treatments. *Open Journal of Pain Medicine*: 4-6.

Hetland, G., E. Johnson, S. V. Bernardshaw, and B. Grinde. 2021. "Can Medicinal Mushrooms Have Prophylactic or Therapeutic Effect against Covid-19 and Its Pneumonic Superinfection and Complicating Inflammation?" *Scandinavian Journal of Immunology* 93, no. 1: e12937. https://doi.org/10.1111/sji.12937.

Hidese, S., S. Ogawa, M. Ota, I. Ishida, Z. Yasukawa, M. Ozeki, and H. Kunugi. 2019. "Effects of L-Theanine Administration on Stress-Related Symptoms and Cognitive Functions in Healthy Adults: A Randomized Controlled Trial." *Nutrients* 11, no. 10: 2362. https://doi.org/10.3390/nu11102362.

Hiedra, R., K. B. Lo, M. Elbashabsheh, et al. 2020. "The Use of IV Vitamin C for Patients with COVID-19: A Case Series." *Expert Review of Anti-infective Therapy* 18, no. 12: 1259-61. https://doi.org/10.1080/14787210.2020.1794819.

Hirayama, M., H. Nishiwaki, T. Hamaguchi, M. Ito, J. Ueyama, T. Maeda, K. Kashihara, Y. Tsuboi, and K. Ohno. 2021. "Intestinal Collinsella May Mitigate Infection and Exacerbation of COVID-19 by Producing Ursodeoxycholate." *PLOS ONE* 16, no. 11: e0260451. https://doi.org/10.1371/journal.pone.0260451.

Hojyo, S., M. Uchida, K. Tanaka, et al. 2020. "How COVID-19 Induces Cytokine Storm with High Mortality." *Inflammation and Regeneration* 40: 37. https://doi.org/10.1186/s41232-020-00146-3.

Holmes, M. D., J. W. Miller, J. Voipio, K. Kaila, and S. Vanhatalo. 2003. "Vagal Nerve Stimulation Induces Intermittent Hypocapnia." *Epilepsia* 44, no. 12: 1588-91. https://doi.org/10.1111/j.0013-9580.2003.19203.x.

Hosp, J. A., A. Dressing, G. Blazhenets, T. Bormann, A. Rau, M. Schwabenland, J. Thurow, et al. 2021. "Cognitive Impairment and Altered Cerebral Glucose Metabolism in the Subacute Stage of COVID-19." *Brain* 144, no. 4: 1263-76. https://doi.org/10.1093/brain/awab009.

Høstmark, A. T., L. Sørensen, and R. Askevold. 1977. "Influence of Sodium Hydroxide on Protein Determination with the Xylene Brilliant Cyanin G Micromethod." *Analytical Biochemistry* 83, no. 2. https://doi.org/10.1016/0003-2697(77)90086-0.

House, R. V., P. T. Thomas, and H. N. Bhargava. 1995. "Comparison of the Hallucinogenic Indole Alkaloids Ibogaine and Harmaline for Potential Immunomodulatory Activity." *Pharmacology* 51, no. 1: 56-65.

Howland, R. H. 2014. "Vagus Nerve Stimulation." *Current Behavioral Neuroscience Reports* 1, no. 2: 64–73. https://doi.org/10.1007/s40473-014-0010-5.

Hu, Di, J. Li, R. Gao, S. Wang, Q. Li, S. Chen, et al. 2021. "Decreased CO2 Levels as Indicators of Possible Mechanical Ventilation-Induced Hyperventilation in COVID-19 Patients: A Retrospective Analysis." *Frontiers in Public Health* 8: 596168.

Hu, Fen Jiao Chen, Hao Chen, Jin Zhu, Chen Wang, Haibin Ni, Jianming Cheng, Xingxing Hu, and Peng Cao. 2021. "Chansu Improves the Respiratory Function of Severe COVID-19 Patients." *Pharmacological Research: Modern Chinese Medicine* 1: 100007. https://doi.org/10.1016/j.prmcm.2021.100007.

Hu, K., J. Patel, C. Swiston, et al. 2022. "Ophthalmic Manifestations of Coronavirus (COVID-19)." StatPearls (online). Treasure Island, Fla.: StatPearls Publishing. Updated May 24, 2022.

Huang, Yong, M. D. Pinto, J. L. Borelli, M. A. Mehrabadi, H. Abrihim, N. Dutt, N. Lambert, et al. 2021. "COVID Symptoms, Symptom Clusters, and Predictors for Becoming a Long-Hauler: Looking for Clarity in the Haze of the Pandemic." medRxiv preprint. https://doi.org/10.1101/2021.03.03.21252086.

Hwang. S. H., I. J. Kang, and S. S. Lim. 2017. "Antidiabetic Effect of Fresh Nopal (*Opuntia ficus-indica*) in Low-Dose Streptozotocin-Induced Diabetic Rats Fed a High-Fat Diet." *Evidence-Based Complementary Alternative Medicine*. https://doi.org/10.1155/2017/4380721.

Hutchinson, Sally Anne. 2016. "The Limbic System, Disease and Homeopathy: How Emotional Stress Affects Our Health." *Homeopathy* 232.

Im, J. H., Y. S. Je, J. Baek, M. H. Chung, H. Y. Kwon, and J. S. Lee. 2020. "Nutritional Status of Patients with COVID-19." *International Journal of Infectious Diseases* 100: 390–93. https://doi.org/10.1016/j.ijid.2020.08.018.

Ingawale, D. K., and S. S. Patel. 2016. "Anti-inflammatory Potential of Hecogenin in Experimental Animals: Possible Involvement of Inflammatory Cytokines and Myeloperoxidase." *Drug Research* 66, no. 12: 644–56. https://doi.org/10.1055/s-0042-113184.

Ingawale, D. K., S. K. Mandlik, and S. S. Patel. 2019. "Anti-inflammatory Potential of Hecogenin on Atopic Dermatitis and Airway Hyper-responsiveness by Regulation of Pro-Inflammatory Cytokines." *Immunopharmacology and Immunotoxicology* 41, no. 2: 327–36.

Ingawale, D. 2020. "Saponins and Sapogenins of Agave with Respect to Diverse Pharmacological Role of Hecogenin." *International Journal of Pharmacy and Pharmaceutical Sciences* 12, no. 2: 1–7. https://doi.org/10.22159/ijpps.2020v12i2.35789.

International New York Times. 2021. "Kambo: The Immunity Boosting Poison Obtained from an Amazonian Frog." *Deccan Herald* (online), January 1, 2021.

Ip, A., J. Ahn, Y. Zhou, et al. 2021. "Hydroxychloroquine in the Treatment of Outpatients with Mildly Symptomatic COVID-19: A Multi-center Observational Study." *BMC Infectious Diseases* 21, no. 72. https://doi.org/10.1186/s12879-021-05773-w.

Jafar, Jalaei, Mehdi Fazeli, Hamid Rajaian, Somayeh Layeghi Ghalehsoukhteh, Alireza Dehghani, and Dominic Winter. 2016. "In vitro Antihistamine-Releasing Activity of a Peptide Derived from Wasp Venom of Vespa orientalis." *Asian Pacific Journal of Tropical Biomedicine* 6, no. 3: 259–64.

Jang, Y., W. J. Lee, G. S. Hong, and W. S. Shim. 2015. "Red Ginseng Extract Blocks Histamine-Dependent Itch by Inhibition of H1R/TRPV1 Pathway in Sensory Neurons." *Journal of Ginseng Research* 39, no. 3: 257–64. https://doi.org/10.1016/j.jgr.2015.01.004.

Jarrott, B., R. Head, K. G. Pringle, E. R. Lumbers, and J. H. Martin. 2022. "'LONG COVID'—A Hypothesis for Understanding the Biological Basis and Pharmacological

Treatment Strategy." *Pharmacology Research & Perspectives* 10, no. 1:e00911. https://doi.org/ 10.1002/prp2.911.

Jeremiah, S. S., K. Miyakawa, T. Morita, Y. Yamaoka, and A. Ryo. 2020. "Potent Antiviral Effect of Silver Nanoparticles on SARS-CoV-2." *Biochemical and Biophysical Research Communications* 533, no. 1: 195–200. https://doi.org/10.1016/j.bbrc.2020.09.018.

Jessen, N. A., A. S. Munk, I. Lundgaard, and M. Nedergaard. 2015. "The Glymphatic System: A Beginner's Guide." *Neurochemical Research* 40, no. 12: 2583–99. https://doi.org/10.1007/s11064-015-1581-6.

Joly, F., L. Galoppin, P. Bordat, H. Cousse, and E. Neuzil. 2000. Calcium and Bicarbonate Ions Mediate the Inhibition of Mast Cell Histamine Release by Avène Spa Water." *Fundamental & Clinical Pharmacology* 14, no. 6: 611–13. https://doi.org/10.1111/j.1472-8206.2000.tb00447.x.

Jung, C. 1968. *Man and His Symbols.* New York: Random House.

Kaminski, P., and K. Katz. 1994. *Flower Essence Repertory.* Nevada City, Calif.: Flower Essence Society.

Kaptchuk, T. J. 1983. *The Web That Has No Weaver: Understanding Chinese Medicine.* New York: Congdon and Weed.

Kasozi, K. I., G. Niedbała, M. Alqarni, G. Zirintunda, F. Ssempijja, S. P. Musinguzi, I. M. Usman, et al. 2020. "Bee Venom—A Potential Complementary Medicine Candidate for SARS-CoV-2 Infections." *Frontiers in Public Health* 8: 594458. https://doi.org/10.3389/fpubh.2020.594458.

Kennedy, D. A., K. Cooley, T. R. Einarson, and D. Seely. 2012. "Objective Assessment of an Ionic Footbath (IonCleanse): Testing Its Ability to Remove Potentially Toxic Elements from the Body." *Journal of Environmental and Public Health* 2012: 258968. https://doi.org/10.1155/2012/258968.

Keppel Hesselink, J. M., T. de Boer, and R. F. Witkamp. 2013. "Palmitoylethanolamide: A Natural Body-Own Anti-inflammatory Agent, Effective and Safe against Influenza and Common Cold." *International Journal of Inflammation* 2013: 151028. https://doi.org/10.1155/2013/151028.

Keta-Cov Research Group. 2021. "Intravenous Ketamine and Progressive Cholangiopathy in COVID-19 Patients." *Journal of Hepatology* 74: 1243–44. https://doi.org/10.1016/j.jhep.2021.02.007.

Khavinson, V, N. Linkova, A. Dyatlova, B. Kuznik, and R. Umnov. 2020. "Peptides: Prospects for Use in the Treatment of COVID-19." *Molecules* 25, no. 19: 4389. https://doi.org/10.3390/molecules25194389.

Khlangwiset, P. G. S. Shephard, F. and Wu. 2011. "Aflatoxins and Growth Impairment: A Review." *Critical Reviews in Toxicology* 41 (no. 9): 740–55.

Kieninger, M., A. Sinning, T. Vadász, M. Gruber, W. Gronwald, et al. 2021. Lower Blood pH as a Strong Prognostic Factor for Fatal Outcomes in Critically Ill COVID-19 Patients at an Intensive Care Unit: A Multivariable Analysis." *PLOS ONE* 16, no. 9: e0258018. https://doi.org/10.1371/journal.pone.0258018.

Kim, N. H., T. H. Park, and M. S. Rhee. 2014. "Enhanced Bactericidal Action of Acidified Sodium Chlorite Caused by the Saturation of Reactants." *Journal of Applied Microbiology* 116, no. 6.

Kindgen-Milles, Detlef, Torsten Feldt, Bjoern Erik Ole Jensen, Thomas Dimski, and Timo Brandenburger. 2022. "Why the Application of IVIG Might Be Beneficial in Patients with COVID-19." *Lancet Respiratory Medicine* 10, no. 2: e15.

Kjellberg, A., A. De Maio, and P. Lindholm. 2020. "Can Hyperbaric Oxygen Safely Serve as an Anti-inflammatory Treatment for COVID-19?" *Medical Hypotheses* 144: 110224. https://doi.org/10.1016/j.mehy.2020.110224.

Klein, R., A. Soung, C. Sissoko, A. Nordvig, P. Canoll, M. Mariani, X. Jiang, et al. 2021.

"COVID-19 Induces Neuroinflammation and Loss of Hippocampal Neurogenesis." Research Square prepint. https://doi.org/10.21203/rs.3.rs-1031824/v1.

Ko, K. H. 2016. "Hominin Interbreeding and the Evolution of Human Variation." *Journal of Biological Research* (Thessaloniki) 23: 17. https://doi.org/10.1186/s40709-016-0054-7.

Kočar, Eva, Tadeja Režen, and Damjana Rozman. 2021. "Cholesterol, Lipoproteins, and COVID-19: Basic Concepts and Clinical Applications." *Biochimica et Biophysica Acta. Molecular and Cell Biology of Lipids* 1866, no. 2: 158849.

Koerber, N., A. Priller, S. Yazici, et al. 2022. "Dynamics of Spike- and Nucleocapsid Specific Immunity during Long-Term Follow-Up and Vaccination of SARS-CoV-2 Convalescents." *Nature Communications* 13, no. 1: 153. https://doi.org/10.1038/s41467-021-27649-y.

Kolahchi, Z., H. Sohrabi, S. Ekrami Nasab, et al. 2021. "Potential Therapeutic Approach of Intravenous Immunoglobulin against COVID-19." *Allergy Asthma and Clinical Immunology* 17, no. 1: 105. https://doi.org/10.1186/s13223-021-00609-3.

Korzeniowska, Anna, Ręka Gabriela, Małgorzata Bilska, and Halina Piecewicz-Szczęsna. 2021. "The Smoker's Paradox during the COVID-19 Pandemic? The Influence of Smoking and Vaping on the Incidence and Course of SARS-CoV-2 Virus Infection as well as Possibility of Using Nicotine in the Treatment of COVID-19 – Review of the Literature." *Przegląd epidemiologiczny* 75, no. 1: 27–44. https://doi.org/10.32394/pe.75.03.

Kritas, S. K., C. E. Gallenga, C. D. Ovidio, G. Ronconi, A. I. Caraffa, E. Toniato, D. Lauritano, and P. Conti. 2018. "Impact of Mold on Mast Cell-Cytokine Immune Response." *Journal of Biological Regulators and Homeostatic Agents* 32, no. 4: 763–68.

Kumaki, Y., M. K. Wandersee, A. J. Smith, Y. Zhou, G. Simmons, N. M. Nelson, K. W. Bailey, et al. 2011. "Inhibition of Severe Acute Respiratory Syndrome Coronavirus Replication in a Lethal SARS-CoV BALB/c Mouse Model by Stinging Nettle Lectin, Urtica dioica Agglutinin." *Antiviral Research* 90, no. 1: 22–32. https://doi.org/10.1016/j.antiviral.2011.02.003.

Kumar, P., M. Kumar, O. Bedi, et al. 2021. "Role of Vitamins and Minerals as Immunity Boosters in COVID-19." *Inflammopharmacology* 29: 1001–16. https://doi.org/10.1007/s10787-021-00826-7.

Kurup, V. P., C. S. Barrios. 2008. "Immunomodulatory Effects of Curcumin in Allergy." *Molecular Nutrition and Food Research* 52, no. 9: 1031–39. https://doi.org/10.1002/mnfr.200700293.

Laccourreye, O., A. Werner, J.-P. Giroud, V. Couloigner, P. Bonfils, and E. Bondon-Guitton. 2015. "Benefits, Limits and Danger of Ephedrine and Pseudoephedrine as Nasal Decongestants." *European Annals of Otorhinolaryngology, Head and Neck Diseases* 132, no. 1: 31–34.

Lavelle, J. N. 2003. *Cracking the Metobolic Code.* San Diego, Calif.: Basic Health Publications.

Lazar, V., L.-M. Ditu, G. G. Pircalabioru, I. Gheorghe, C. Curutiu, A. M. Holban, A. Picu, L. Petcu, and M. C. Chifiriuc. 2018. "Aspects of Gut Microbiota and Immune System Interactions in Infectious Diseases, Immunopathology, and Cancer." *Frontiers in Immunology* 9: 1830. https://doi.org/10.3389/fimmu.2018.01830.

Lehrer, S., and P. H. Rheinstein. 2020. "Ivermectin Docks to the SARS-CoV-2 Spike Receptor-Binding Domain Attached to ACE2." *In Vivo* 34, no. 5: 3023–26. https://doi.org/10.21873/invivo.12134.

Leimer, N., X. Wu, Y. Imai, M. Morrissette, N. Pitt, Q. Favre-Godal, A. Iinishi, et al. 2021. "A Selective Antibiotic for Lyme Disease." *Cell* 184, no. 21: 5405–18:e16. https://doi.org/10.1016/j.cell.2021.09.011.

Lein, Peiting. 2021. "Coronavirus Recovery: Breathing Exercises." Johns Hopkins Medicine (online). May 11, 2021.

Lenze, E. J., C. Mattar, C. F. Zorumski, et al. 2020. "Fluvoxamine vs Placebo and Clinical Deterioration in Outpatients with Symptomatic COVID-19: A Randomized Clinical Trial." *JAMA* 324, no. 22: 2292–200. https://doi.org/10.1001/jama.2020.22760.

Lerner, A. M., S. H. Beqaj, R. G. Deeter, H. J. Dworkin, M. Zervos, C. H. Chang, J. T. Fitzgerald, J. Goldstein, and W. O'Neill. 2002. "A Six-Month Trial of Valacyclovir in the Epstein-Barr Virus Subset of Chronic Fatigue Syndrome: Improvement in Left Ventricular Function." *Drugs Today* (Barc) 38, no. 8: 549–61.

Li, Y., Z. Wang, N. Lian, Y. Wang, W. Zheng, K. Xie. 2021. "Molecular Hydrogen: A Promising Adjunctive Strategy for the Treatment of the COVID-19." *Frontiers in Medicine (Lausanne)* 8:671215. https://doi.org/10.3389/fmed.2021.671215.

Li, L. C., H. M. Piao, M. Y. Zheng, Z. H. Lin, G. Li, and G. H. Yan. 2016. "Sesamin Attenuates Mast Cell-Mediated Allergic Responses by Suppressing the Activation of p38 and Nuclear Factor-κB." *Molecular Medicine Reports* 13, no. 1: 536–42. https://doi.org/10.3892/mmr.2015.4546.

Liang, J., J. Chen, Z. Tan, J. Peng, X. Zheng, K. Nishiura, et al. 2013. Extracts of Medicinal Herb Sanguisorba officinalis Inhibit the Entry of Human Immunodeficiency Virus Type One." *Journal of Food and Drug Analysis* 21: S52–58. https://doi.org/10.1016/j.jfda.2013.09.034.

Lin, Z., W. Phyu, Z. Phyu, et al. 2021 "The Role of Steroids in the Management of COVID-19 Infection." *Cureus* 13, no. 8: e16841. https://doi.org/10.7759/cureus.16841.

Lind, S. E. 2021. "Phosphatidylserine Is an Overlooked Mediator of COVID-19 Thromboinflammation." *Heliyon* 7, no. 1: e06033. https://doi.org/10.1016/j.heliyon.2021.e06033.

Lippi, G., A. M. South, and B. M. Henry. 2020. "Electrolyte Imbalances in Patients with Severe Coronavirus Disease 2019 (COVID-19)." *Annals of Clinical Biochemistry* 57, no. 3: 262–65. https://doi.org/10.1177/0004563220922255.

Liu, Q., J. W. Y. Mak, Q. Su, et al. 2022. "Gut Microbiota Dynamics in a Prospective Cohort of Patients with Post-Acute COVID-19 Syndrome." *Gut* 71: 544–52.

Liu, Y., A. H. Sawalha, Q. Lu. 2021. "COVID-19 and Autoimmune Diseases." *Current Opinion in Rheumatology* 33, no. 2: 155–62. https://doi.org/10.1097/BOR.0000000000000776.

Lopez-Leon, S., T. Wegman-Ostrosky, C. Perelman, et al. 2021. "More Than 50 Long-Term Effects of COVID-19: A Systematic Review and Meta-Analysis." *Scientific Reports* 11, no. 1: 16144. https://doi.org/10.1038/s41598-021-95565-8.

Loretelli, C., A. Abdelsalam, F. D'Addio, M. Ben Nasr, E. Assi, V. Usuelli, A. Maestroni, A. J. Seelam, E. Ippolito, S. Di Maggio, L. Loreggian, D. Radovanovic, C. Vanetti, J. Yang, B. El Essawy, A. Rossi et al. 2021. "PD-1 Blockade Counteracts Post-COVID-19 Immune Abnormalities and Stimulates the Anti-SARS-CoV-2 Immune Response." *JCI Insight* 6, no. 24. https://doi.org/10.1172/jci.insight.146701.

Lubell, Jeffrey. 2021. "Why Does High-Dose Thiamine Relieve Fatigue in Individuals with Diverse Conditions? Hypotheses Grounded in Thiamine's Role as a Carbonic Anhydrase Inhibitor." EDS Perspectives (online), January 10, 2021.

Luliano, A. D., J. M. Brunkard, T. K. Boehmer, et al. 2022. "Trends in Disease Severity and Health Care Utilization during the Early Omicron Variant Period Compared with Previous SARS-CoV-2 High Transmission Periods—United States, December 2020–January 2022." *Morbidity and Mortality Weekly Report* 71, no. 4: 146–52.

Ma, C., Y. Cong, and H. Zhang. 2020. "COVID-19 and the Digestive System." American Journal of Gastroenterology 115, no. 7: 1003–1006. https://doi.org/10.14309/ajg.0000000000000691.

MaassenVanDenBrink, A., T. de Vries, and A. H. J. Danser. 2020. "Headache Medication and the COVID-19 Pandemic." *Journal of Headache and Pain* 21, no. 38. https://doi.org/10.1186/s10194-020-01106-5.

MacDonald, Alan B. 2016. "Mutilple Sclerosis Is a Parasitosis." Medical lecture. London, England. Available on YouTube.

Mackay, Angus. 2021. "A Paradigm for Post-Covid-19 Fatigue Syndrome Analogous to ME/CFS." *Frontiers in Neurology* 12. https://doi.org/10.3389/fneur.2021.701419.

Mahendran, A. S. K., Y. S. Lim, C.-M. Fang, H.-S. Loh, and C. F. Le. 2020. "The Potential of Antiviral Peptides as COVID-19 Therapeutics." *Frontiers in Pharmacology* 11: 575444. https://doi.org/10.3389/fphar.2020.575444.

Mahima, A. Rahal, R. Deb, S. K. Latheef, H. Abdul Samad, R. Tiwari, A. K. Verma, A. Kumar, and K. Dhama. 2012. "Immunomodulatory and Therapeutic Potentials of Herbal, Traditional/Indigenous and Ethnoveterinary Medicines." *Pakistan Journal of Biological Science* 15, no. 16: 754–74. https://doi.org/10.3923/pjbs.2012.754.774.

Mahmud, R., M. M. Rahman, I. Alam, et al. 2021. "Ivermectin in Combination with Doxycycline for Treating COVID-19 Symptoms: A Randomized Trial." *Journal of International Medical Research* 49, no. 5. https://doi.org/10.1177/03000605211013550.

Malayala, S. V., and A. Raza. 2020. "A Case of COVID-19-Induced Vestibular Neuritis." *Cureus* 12, no. 6: e8918. https://doi.org/10.7759/cureus.8918.

Malone, R. W., P. Tisdall, P. Fremont-Smith, et al. 2021. "COVID-19: Famotidine, Histamine, Mast Cells, and Mechanisms." *Frontiers in Pharmacology* 12. https://doi.org/10.3389/fphar.2021.633680.

Mamedov, Tarlan, İrem Gürbüzaslan, Merve Ilgin, Damla Yuksel, Gunay Mammadova, Aykut Ozkul, and Gulnara Hasanova. 2021. "High Level Production and Characterization of Truncated Human Angiotensin Converting Enzyme 2 in Nicotiana benthamiana Plant as a Potential Therapeutic Target in COVID-19." bioRxiv preprint. https://doi.org/10.1101/2021.05.17.444533.

Mansanguan, S., P. Charunwatthana, W. Piyaphanee, W. Dechkhajorn, A. Poolcharoen, and C. Mansanguan. 2022. "Cardiovascular Manifestation of the BNT162b2 mRNA COVID-19 Vaccine in Adolescents." *Tropical Medicine and Infectious Disease* 7, no. 8: 196. https://doi.org/10.3390/tropicalmed7080196.

Marx, V. 2021. "Scientists Set Out to Connect the Dots on Long COVID." *Nature Methods* 18: 449–53. https://doi.org/10.1038/s41592-021-01145-z.

Masana, L., E. Correig, D. Ibarretxe, et al. 2021. "Low HDL and High Triglycerides Predict COVID-19 Severity." *Scientific Reports* 11: 7217. https://doi.org/10.1038/s41598-021-86747-5.

Massey, Daisy, Diana Berrent, and Harlan Krumholz. 2021. "Breakthrough Symptomatic COVID-19 Infections Leading to Long Covid: Report from Long Covid Facebook Group Poll." medRxiv preprint. https://doi.org/10.1101/2021.07.23.21261030.

Mateos-Aparicio, Pedro, and Antonio Rodríguez-Moreno. 2019. "The Impact of Studying Brain Plasticity." *Frontiers in Cellular Neuroscience* 13: 66. https://doi.org/10.3389/fncel.2019.00066.

May, B. C., and K. H. Gallivan. 2022. "Levocetirizine and Montelukast in the COVID-19 Treatment Paradigm." *International Immunopharmacology* 103, no. 108412.

Medina-Enríquez, M. M., S. Lopez-León, J. A. Carlos-Escalante, et al. 2020. "ACE2: The Molecular Doorway to SARS-CoV-2." *Cell and Bioscience* 10: 148. https://doi.org/10.1186/s13578-020-00519-8.

Mehandru, S., and M. Merad. 2022. "Pathological Sequelae of Long-Haul COVID. *Nature Immunology* 23: 194–202. https://doi.org/10.1038/s41590-021-01104-y.

Mergenthaler, P., U. Lindauer, G. A. Dienel, and A. Meisel. 2013. "Sugar for the Brain:

The Role of Glucose in Physiological and Pathological Brain Function." *Trends in Neurosciences* 36, no. 10: 587–97. https://doi.org/10.1016/j.tins.2013.07.001.

Micol, Vicente, Nuria Caturla, Laura Pérez-Fons, Vicente Más, Luis Pérez, and Amparo Estepa. 2005. "The Olive Leaf Extract Exhibits Antiviral Activity against Viral Haemorrhagic Septicaemia Rhabdovirus (VHSV)." *Antiviral Research* 66, no. 2–3: 129–36.

Miller, R., A. R. Wentzel, and G. A. Richards. 2020. "COVID-19: NAD+ Deficiency May Predispose the Aged, Obese and Type2 Diabetics to Mortality through Its Effect on SIRT1 Activity." *Medical Hypotheses* 144: 110044. https://doi.org/10.1016/j.mehy.2020.110044.

Mir, Mudasir A., Sheikh Mansoor, Abida Bhat, Muneeb U. Rehman, Ajaz Ahmad, and Parvaiz Ahmad. 2020. "Lysosomotropic Properties of Sodium Bicarbonate and Covid-19." *Farmacia* 68, no. 5.

Misra, A. K., S. K. Varma, and R. Kumar. 2018. "Anti-inflammatory Effect of an Extract of Agave americana on Experimental Animals." *Pharmacognosy Research* 10, no. 1: 104–8. https://doi.org/10.4103/pr.pr_64_17.

Mlcek, J., T. Jurikova, S. Skrovankova, and J. Sochor. 2016. "Quercetin and Its Anti-allergic Immune Response." *Molecules* 21, no. 5: 623. https://doi.org/10.3390/molecules21050623.

Mock, S. E., and S. M. Arai. 2011. "Childhood Trauma and Chronic Illness in Adulthood: Mental Health and Socioeconomic Status as Explanatory Factors and Buffers." *Frontiers in Psychology* 1: 246. https://doi.org/10.3389/fpsyg.2010.00246.

Montefusco, L., M. Ben Nasr, F. D'Addio, et al. 2021. "Acute and Long-Term Disruption of Glycometabolic Control after SARS-CoV-2 Infection." *Nature Metabolism* 3: 774–85. https://doi.org/10.1038/s42255-021-00407-6.

Monterrosas-Brisson, N., M. L. Ocampo, E. Jiménez-Ferrer, et al. 2013. "Anti-inflammatory Activity of Different Agave Plants and the Compound Cantalasaponin-1. *Molecules* 18, no. 7: 8136–46. https://doi.org/10.3390/molecules18078136.

Moosavi, M. 2017. "Bentonite Clay as a Natural Remedy: A Brief Review." *Iranian Journal of Public Health* 46, no. 9: 1176–83.

Moses, T., K. K. Papadopoulou, and A. Osbourn. 2014. "Metabolic and Functional Diversity of Saponins, Biosynthetic Intermediates and Semi-synthetic Derivatives." *Critical Reviews in Biochemistry and Molecular Biology* 49, no. 6: 439–62. https://doi.org/10.3109/10409238.2014.953628.

Moskowitz, J. M. 2018. "Scientific Evidence of Harm from Cell Phone Radiation: Two Years Research." *Electromagnetic Radiation Safety*, August 8, 2018.

Mousavi, S. A., K. Heydari, H. Mehravaran, M. Saeedi, R. Alizadeh-Navaei, A. Hedayatizadeh-Omran, and A. Shamshirian. 2022. "Melatonin Effects on Sleep Quality and Outcomes of COVID-19 Patients: An Open-Label, Randomized, Controlled Trial. *Journal of Medical Virology* 94, no. 1: 263–71. https://doi.org/10.1002/jmv.27312.

Mulle, J. G., W. G. Sharp, and J. F. Cubells. 2013. "The Gut Microbiome: A New Frontier in Autism Research." *Current Psychiatry Reports* 15, no. 2.

Müller, C., N. Karl, J. Ziebuhr, and S. Pleschka. 2016. "D, L-lysine Acetylsalicylate + Glycine Impairs Coronavirus Replication." *Journal of Antivirals and Antiretrovirals* 8, no. 4: 142–50. https://doi.org/10.4172/jaa.1000151.

Mulrow, C., V. Lawrence, B. Jacobs, et al. 2000. "Milk Thistle: Effects on Liver Disease and Cirrhosis and Clinical Adverse Effects: Summary." In *AHRQ Evidence Report Summaries*. Rockville, Md.: Agency for Healthcare Research and Quality, 1998–2005.

Murphy, William J., and Dan L. Longo. 2022. "A Possible Role for Anti-idiotype Antibodies in SARS-CoV-2 Infection and Vaccination." *New England*

Journal of Medicine 386: 394–96. https://doi.org/10.1056/NEJMcibr2113694.

Musthafa, M. S., A. R. Jawahar Ali, A. R. Hyder Ali, et al. 2016. "Effect of Shilajit Enriched Diet on Immunity, Antioxidants, and Disease Resistance in Macrobrachium rosenbergii (de Man) against Aeromonas hydrophila." *Fish and Shellfish Immunology* 57: 293–300. https://doi.org/10.1016/j.fsi.2016.08.033.

Myss, C. 1996. *Anatomy of the Spirit: The Seven Stages of Power and Healing.* Walpole, N.H.: Stillpoint.

Nabatov, A. A., G. Pollakis, T. Linnemann, W. A. Paxton, and M. P. de Baar. 2007. "Statins Disrupt CCR5 and RANTES Expression Levels in CD4(+) T Lymphocytes In Vitro and Preferentially Decrease Infection of R5 versus X4 HIV-1." *PLOS ONE* 2, no. 5: e470. https://doi.org/10.1371/journal.pone.0000470.

Naidu, Sindhu B., Amar J. Shah, Anita Saigal, Colette Smith, Simon E. Brill, James Goldring, John R. Hurst, Hannah Jarvis, Marc Lipman, and Swapna Mandal. 2021. "The High Mental Health Burden of 'Long COVID' and Its Association with On-going Physical and Respiratory Symptoms in All Adults Discharged from Hospital." *European Respiratory Journal.* https://doi.org/10.1183/13993003.04364-2020.

Nakamura, S., R. Hisamura, S. Shimoda, I. Shibuya, and K. Tsubota. 2014. "Fasting Mitigates Immediate Hypersensitivity: A Pivotal Role of Endogenous D-beta-hydroxybutyrate." *Nutrition and Metabolism* 11: 40. https://doi.org/10.1186/1743-7075-11-40.

Nalbandian, A., K. Sehgal, A. Gupta, et al. 2021. "Post-Acute COVID-19 Syndrome." *Nature Medicine* 27: 601–15. https://doi.org/10.1038/s41591-021-01283-z.

Navegantes, K. C., R. de Souza Gomes, P. A. T. Pereira, et al. 2017. "Immune Modulation of Some Autoimmune Diseases: The Critical Role of Macrophages and Neutrophils in the Innate and Adaptive Immunity." *Journal of Translational Medicine* 15, no. 1: 36. https://doi.org/10.1186/s12967-017-1141-8.

Ng, T. P. M. Lim, M. Niti, and S. Collinson. 2012. "Long Term Digital Phone Use and Cognitive Decline in the Elderly." *Bioelectromagnetics* 33, no. 2 (February): 176–85.

Nguyen, A. A., S. B. Habiballah, C. D. Platt, R. S. Geha, J. S. Chou, and D. R. McDonald. 2020. "Immunoglobulins in the Treatment of COVID-19 Infection: Proceed with Caution!" *Clinical Immunology* 216: 108459. https://doi.org/10.1016/j.clim.2020.108459.

Niciu, M. J., I. D. Henter, D. A. Luckenbaugh, C. A. Zarate Jr., and D. S. Charney. 2014. "Glutamate Receptor Antagonists as Fast-Acting Therapeutic Alternatives for the Treatment of Depression: Ketamine and Other Compounds." *Annual Review of Pharmacology and Toxicology* 54: 119–39. https://doi.org/10.1146/annurev-pharmtox-011613-135950.

Noels, H., and C. Weber. 2010. "Fractalkine as an Important Target of Aspirin in the Prevention of Atherogenesis." *Cardiovascular Drugs and Therapy* 24: 1–3. https://doi.org/10.1007/s10557-009-6213-4

Nowaczewska, M., M. Wiciński, and W. Kaźmierczak. 2020. "The Ambiguous Role of Caffeine in Migraine Headache: From Trigger to Treatment." *Nutrients* 12, no. 8: 2259. https://doi.org/10.3390/nu12082259.

Nugent, Nicole R., Amy Goldberg, and Monica Uddin. 2016. "Topical Review: The Emerging Field of Epigenetics: Informing Models of Pediatric Trauma and Physical Health." *Journal of Pediatric Psychology* 41, no. 1: 55–64. https://doi.org/10.1093/jpepsy/jsv018.

Nurek, Martine, C. Rayner, A. Freyer, S. Taylor, L. Järte, N. MacDermott, B. C. Delaney, and Delphi panellists. 2021. "Recommendations for the Recognition, Diagnosis, and Management of Long COVID: A Delphi Study." *British Journal of General Practice* 71, no. 712: e815–e825. https://doi.org/10.3399/BJGP.2021.0265.

Ogata, Alana F., Chi-An Cheng, Michaël Desjardins, Yasmeen Senussi, Amy C. Sherman, Megan Powell, Lewis Novack, Salena Von, Xiaofang Li, Lindsey R. Baden, and David R. Walt. 2022. "Circulating Severe Acute Respiratory Syndrome Coronavirus 2 (SARS-CoV-2) Vaccine Antigen Detected in the Plasma of mRNA-1273 Vaccine Recipients." *Clinical Infectious Diseases* 74, no. 4: 715–18. https://doi.org/10.1093/cid/ciab465.

Ogata, Norio, and Takanori Miura. 2021. "Inhibition of the Binding of Variants of SARS-CoV-2. Coronavirus Spike Protein to a Human Receptor by Chlorine Dioxide." *Annals of Pharmacology and Pharmaceutics* 5, no. 5: 1195.

Ostuzzi, G., D. Papola, C. Gastaldon, et al. 2020. "Safety of Psychotropic Medications in People with COVID-19: Evidence Review and Practical Recommendations." *BMC Medicine* 18: 215. https://doi.org/10.1186/s12916-020-01685-9.

Otterbein, L., F. Bach, J. Alam, et al. 2000. "Carbon Monoxide Has Anti-inflammatory Effects Involving the Mitogen-Activated Protein Kinase Pathway." *Nature Medicine* 6: 422–28. https://doi.org/10.1038/74680.

Ou, L., B. Song, H. Liang, et al. 2016. "Toxicity of Graphene-Family Nanoparticles: A General Review of the Origins and Mechanisms." *Particle and Fibre Toxicology* 13: 57. https://doi.org/10.1186/s12989-016-0168-y.

Pairo-Castineira, E., S. Clohisey, L. Klaric, et al. 2021. "Genetic Mechanisms of Critical Illness in COVID-19." *Nature* 591: 92–98. https://doi.org/10.1038/s41586-020-03065-y.

Pal, Rimesh, Mainak Banerjee, and Sanjay K Bhadada. 2020. "Cortisol Concentrations and Mortality from COVID-19." *Lancet Diabetes & Endocrinology* 8, no. 10: 809.

Palmos, Alish B., Vincent Millischer, David K. Menon, Timothy R. Nicholson, Leonie Taams, Benedict Michael, COVID Clinical Neuroscience Study Consortium, Christopher Hübel, and Gerome Breen. 2022. "Proteome-Wide Mendelian Randomization Identifies Causal Links between Blood Proteins and Severe COVID-19." *PLOS Genetics* 18, no. 3: e1010042. https://doi.org/10.1371/journal.pgen.1010042.

Panahi, Yasin, Masoomeh Dadkhah, Sahand Talei, Zahra Gharari, Vahid Asghariazar, Arash Abdolmaleki, Somayeh Matin, and Soheila Molaei. 2022. "Can Anti-parasitic Drugs Help Control COVID-19?" *Future Virology* 17, no. 5: 315–39.

Papadopoulou, Areti, Hanan Musa, Mathura Sivaganesan, David McCoy, Panos Deloukas, and Eirini Marouli. 2021. "COVID-19 Susceptibility Variants Associate with Blood Clots, Thrombophlebitis and Circulatory Diseases." *PLOS ONE* 16, no. 9: e0256988. https://doi.org/10.1371/journal.pone.0256988.

Park, H. A. 2021. "Fruit Intake to Prevent and Control Hypertension and Diabetes." *Korean Journal of Family Medicine* 42, no. 1: 9–16. https://doi.org/10.4082/kjfm.20.0225.

Parkitny, L., J. Younger. 2017. "Reduced Pro-inflammatory Cytokines after Eight Weeks of Low-Dose Naltrexone for Fibromyalgia." *Biomedicines* 5, no. 2:16. https://doi.org/10.3390/biomedicines5020016.

Parmenter, J. R., and B. Uhrenholdt. 1976. "Effects of Smoke on Pathogens and Other Fungi." In *Proceedings, Tall Timbers Fire Ecology and Fire Land Management Symposium,* no. 14, 299–304. Tallahassee, Fla.: Tall Timbers Research Station.

Patel, S., J. H. Miao, E. Yetiskul, et al. 2022. "Physiology, Carbon Dioxide Retention." StatPearls (online). Treasure Island, Fla.: StatPearls Publishing. Updated January 4, 2022.

Patne, T., J. Mahore, and P. Tokmurke. 2020. "Inhalation of Essential Oils: Could Be Adjuvant Therapeutic Strategy for COVID-19." *International Journal of Pharmaceutical Sciences and Research* 11, no. 9: 4095–103. https://doi.org/10.13040/IJPSR.0975-8232.

Patterson, Bruce. 2022a. "Dr Bruce Patterson Presentation at Georgetown University on Diagnosis and Treatment of Long Haul Covid" (YouTube). Feb 2022

———. 2022b. "Long Covid Discussion with Dr. Bruce Patterson." Dr. Mobeen Medical Lectures (YouTube). January 31, 2022.

Patterson, B. K., E. B. Francisco, R. Yogendra, E. Long, A. Pise, H. Rodrigues, E. Hall, et al. 2022a. "Persistence of SARS CoV-2 S1 Protein in CD16+ Monocytes in Post-Acute Sequelae of COVID-19 (PASC) up to 15 Months Post-infection." *Frontiers in Immunology* 12: 746021. https://doi.org/10.3389/fimmu.2021.746021.

Patterson, Bruce K., Edgar B. Francisco, Ram Yogendra, Emily Long, Amruta Pise, Christopher Beaty, Eric Osgood, et al. 2022b. "SARS-CoV-2 S1 Protein Persistence in SARS-CoV-2 Negative Post-Vaccination Individuals with Long COVID/ PASC-Like Symptoms." Research square preprint (version 1). https://doi.org/10.21203/rs.3.rs-1844677/v1.

Patterson, Bruce, Ram Yogendra, Jose Guevara-Coto, Rodrigo Mora-Rodriguez, Eric Osgood, John Bream, Purvi Parikh, Mark Kreimer, Gary Kaplan, and Michal Zgoda. 2022c. "Targeting the Monocytic-Endothelial-Platelet Axis with Maraviroc and Pravastatin as a Therapeutic Option to Treat Long COVID/Post-Acute Sequelae of COVID (PASC)." Research Square preprint. https://doi.org/10.21203/rs.3.rs-1344323/v1.

Paul, Bindu D., Marian D. Lemle, Anthony L. Komaroff, and Solomon H. Snyder. 2021. "Redox Imbalance Links COVID-19 and Myalgic Encephalomyelitis/Chronic Fatigue Syndrome." *Proceedings of the National Academy of Sciences* 118, no. 34: e2024358118. https://doi.org/10.1073/pnas.2024358118.

Peng, Longping, Dong Yidan, Fan Hua, Cao Min, Wu Qiong, Wang Yi, Zhou Chang, Li Shuchun, Zhao Cheng, and Wang Youhua. 2020. "Traditional Chinese Medicine Regulating Lymphangiogenesis: A Literature Review." *Frontiers in Pharmacology* 11: 1259.

Phillips, Steven, and Michelle A. Williams. 2021. "Confronting Our Next National Health Disaster—Long-Haul Covid." *New England Journal of Medicine* 385: 577–79 https://doi.org/10.1056/NEJMp2109285.

Pizzorno J. 2014. "Mitochondria: Fundamental to Life and Health." *Integrative Medicine* 13, no. 2: 8–15.

Pogoda, J. M., N. B. Gross, X. Arakaki, A. N. Fonteh, R. P. Cowan, and M. G. Harrington. 2016. "Severe Headache or Migraine History Is Inversely Correlated with Dietary Sodium Intake: NHANES 1999–2004." *Headache* 56, no. 4: 688–98. https://doi.org/10.1111/head.12792.

Porges, S. W. 2009. "The Polyvagal Theory: New Insights into Adaptive Reactions of the Autonomic Nervous System." *Cleveland Clinic Journal of Medicine* 76, suppl. 2: S86–90. https://doi.org/10.3949/ccjm.76.s2.17.

Poudel, S., J. Quinonez, J. Choudhari, et al. 2021. "Medical Cannabis, Headaches, and Migraines: A Review of the Current Literature." *Cureus* 13, no. 8: e17407. https://doi.org/10.7759/cureus.17407.

Pretorius, E., M. Vlok, C. Venter, et al. 2021. "Persistent Clotting Protein Pathology in Long COVID/Post-Acute Sequelae of COVID-19 (PASC) Is Accompanied by Increased Levels of Antiplasmin." *Cardiovascular Diabetology* 20: 172. https://doi.org/10.1186/s12933-021-01359-7.

Puttaswamy, H., H. G. Gowtham, M. D. Ojha, et al. 2020. "In Silico Studies Evidenced the Role of Structurally Diverse Plant Secondary Metabolites in Reducing SARS-CoV-2 Pathogenesis." *Scientific Reports* 10: 20584. https://doi.org/10.1038/s41598-020-77602-0.

Quinney, M. 2020. "The COVID-19 Recovery Must Focus on Nature." World Ecnomic Forum (online). April 14, 2020.

Rabagliati, R, N. Rodríguez, C. Núñez, A. Huete, S. Bravo, and P. Garcia. 2021. "COVID-19–Associated Mold Infection in Critically Ill Patients, Chile." *Emerging Infectious Diseases* 27, no. 5: 1454–56. https://doi.org/10.3201/eid2705.204412.

Raj, S. R., A. C. Arnold, A. Barboi, et al. 2021. "Long-COVID Postural Tachycardia Syndrome: An American Autonomic Society Statement." *Clinical Autonomic Research* 31, no. 3: 365–68. https://doi.org/10.1007/s10286-021-00798-2.

Rajmohan, V., and E. Mohandas. 2007. "The Limbic System." *Indian Journal of Psychiatry* 49, no. 2: 132–39. https://doi.org/10.4103/0019-5545.33264.

Ramachandran, L., V. S. Dontaraju, J. Troyer, J. Sahota. 2022. "New Onset Systemic Lupus Erythematosus after COVID-19 Infection: A Case Report. *AME Case Reports* 6, no. 14. https://doi.org/10.21037/acr-21-55.

Ramdani, L. H., and K. Bachari. 2020. "Potential Therapeutic Effects of Resveratrol against SARS-CoV-2." *Acta Virologica* 64, no. 3: 276–80. https://doi.org/10.4149/av_2020_309.

Rathe, M., K. Müller, P. T. Sangild, and S. Husby. 2014. "Clinical Applications of Bovine Colostrum Therapy: A Systematic Review." *Nutrition Reviews* 72, no. 4: 237–54. https://doi.org/10.1111/nure.12089.

Rawat, Aarti, and Rakesh Roshan Mali. 2013. "Phytochemical Properties and Pharmcological Activities of Nicotiana tabacum: A Review." *Indian Journal of Pharmaceutical and Biological Research* 1, no. 2: 74–82.

Ray, S. C., B. Baban, M. A. Tucker, A. J. Seaton, K. C. Chang, E. C. Mannon, J. Sun, et al. 2018. "Oral NaHCO3 Activates a Splenic Anti-inflammatory Pathway: Evidence That Cholinergic Signals Are Transmitted via Mesothelial Cells." *Journal of Immunology* 200: 3568–86. https://doi.org/10.4049/jimmunol.1701605.

Redwine, L. S., C. B. Pert, J. D. Rone, et al. 1999. "Peptide T blocks GP120/CCR5 Chemokine Receptor-Mediated Chemotaxis." *Clinical Immunology* 93, no. 2: 124–31. https://doi.org/10.1006/clim.1999.4771.

Regidor, P. A. 2020. "Covid-19 Management with Inflammation Resolving Mediators? Perspectives and Potential." *Medical Hypotheses* 142: 109813. https://doi.org/10.1016/j.mehy.2020.109813.

Reyes, A. Z., K. A. Hu, J. Teperman, et al. 2021. "Anti-inflammatory Therapy for COVID-19 Infection: The Case for Colchicine." *Annals of the Rheumatic Diseases* 80: 550–57.

Risner, K. H., K. V. Tieu, Y. Wang, et al. 2020. "Maraviroc Inhibits SARS-CoV-2 Multiplication and S-Protein Mediated Cell Fusion in Cell Culture." bioRxiv preprint. https://doi.org/10.1101/2020.08.12.246389.

Rojas, M., Y. Rodríguez, Y. Acosta-Ampudia, et al. 2022. "Autoimmunity Is a Hallmark of Post-COVID Syndrome." *Journal of Translational Medicine* 20, no. 129. https://doi.org/10.1186/s12967-022-03328-4.

Roner, M. R., J. Sprayberry, M. Spinks, and S. Dhanji. 2007. "Antiviral Activity Obtained from Aqueous Extracts of the Chilean Soapbark Tree (Quillaja saponaria Molina)." *Journal of General Virology* 88 (Pt 1): 275–85. https://doi.org/ 10.1099/vir.0.82321-0.

Rosas-Taraco, A., E. Sanchez, S. Garcia, N. Heredia, and D. Bhatnagar. 2011. "Extracts of Agave Americana Inhibit Aflatoxin Production in Aspergillus parasiticus." *World Mycotoxin Journal* 4, no. 1: 37–42.

Rowen, Robert. 2003. "Carnivore Dramatically Stimulates Our Immune System to Treat or Cure About Any Condition That Would Benefit from a Strong Immune System." Innovative Medicine website, January 8, 2013.

Rubik, Beverly, and Robert R. Brown. 2021. "Evidence for a Connection between Coronavirus Disease-19 and Exposure to Radiofrequency Radiation from Wireless Communications Including 5G." *Journal of Clinical and Translational Research* 7, no. 5: 666–81.

Russo, M. A., D. M. Santarelli, and D. O'Rourke. 2017. "The Physiological Effects of Slow

Breathing in the Healthy Human." *Breathe* (Sheff) 13, no. 4: 298–309. https://doi .org/10.1183/20734735.009817.

Sabaratnam, V., W. Kah-Hui, M. Naidu, and P. R. David. 2013. "Neuronal Health— Can Culinary and Medicinal Mushrooms Help?" *Journal of Traditional and Complementary Medicine* 3, no. 1: 62–68. https://doi.org/10.4103/2225-4110.106549.

Saeedi-Boroujeni, A., and M. R. Mahmoudian-Sani. 2021. "Anti-inflammatory Potential of Quercetin in COVID-19 Treatment." *Journal of Inflammation* 18: 3. https://doi .org/10.1186/s12950-021-00268-6.

Safavi, Farinaz, Lindsey Gustafson, Brian Walitt, Tanya Lehky, Sara Dehbashi, Amanda Wiebold, Yair Mina, Susan Shin, Baohan Pan, Michael Polydefkis, et al. 2022. "Neuropathic Symptoms with SARS-CoV-2 Vaccination." medRxiv preprint. https:// doi.org/ 10.1101/2022.05.16.22274439.

Sagar, S., A. K. Rathinavel, W. E. Lutz, et al. 2020. "Bromelain Inhibits SARS-CoV-2 Infection in VeroE6 Cells." bioRxiv preprint. https://doi .org/10.1101/2020.09.16.297366.

Saggam, A., K. Limgaokar, S. Borse, P. Chavan-Gautam, S. Dixit, G. Tillu, and B. Patwardhan. 2021. "Withania somnifera (L.) Dunal: Opportunity for Clinical Repurposing in COVID-19 Management." *Frontiers in Pharmacology* 12: 623795. https://doi.org/10.3389/fphar.2021.623795.

Sánchez, E., N. Heredia, and S. García. 2005. "Inhibition of Growth and Mycotoxin Production of Aspergillus flavus and Aspergillus parasiticus by Extracts of Agave Species." *International Journal of Food Microbiology* 98, no. 3: 271–79. https://doi .org/10.1016/j.ijfoodmicro.2004.07.009.

Sartori, H. E. 1986. "Lithium Orotate in the Treatment of Alcoholism and Related Conditions." *Alcohol* 3, no. 2: 97–100. https://doi.org/10.1016/0741-8329(86)90018-2.

Sasaki-Otomaru, A., Y. Sakuma, Y. Mochizuki, S. Ishida, Y. Kanoya, and C. Sato. 2011. "Effect of Regular Gum Chewing on Levels of Anxiety, Mood, and Fatigue in Healthy Young Adults." *Clinical Practice & Epidemiology in Mental Health* 7: 133–39. https://doi.org/10.2174/1745017901107010133.

Sayana, S., and H. Khanlou. 2009. "Maraviroc: A New CCR5 Antagonist." *Expert Review of Anti-infective Therapy* 7, no. 1: 9–19. https://doi.org/10.1586/14787210.7.1.9.

Schäfer, G., and C. H. Kaschula. 2014. "The Immunomodulation and Anti-inflammatory Effects of Garlic Organosulfur Compounds in Cancer Chemoprevention." *Anticancer Agents in Medicinal Chemistry* 14, no. 2: 233–40. https://doi.org/10.2174 /18715206113136660370.

Schnedl, W. J., M. Schenk, S. Lackner, D. Enko, H. Mangge, and F. Forster. 2019. "Diamine Oxidase Supplementation Improves Symptoms in Patients with Histamine Intolerance." *Food Science and Biotechnology* 28, no. 6: 1779–84. https://doi .org/10.1007/s10068-019-00627-3.

Sears, M. E. 2013. "Chelation: Harnessing and Enhancing Heavy Metal Detoxification—A Review." *Scientific World Journal*: 219840. https://doi.org/10.1155/2013/219840.

Seneff, Stephanie, Anthony M. Kyriakopoulos, Greg Nigh, and Peter A. Mccullough. 2022. "SARS-CoV-2 Spike Protein in the Pathogenesis of Prion-like Diseases." *Authorea*. https://doi.org/10.22541/au.166069342.27133443/v1.

Sepah, Y., L. Samad, A. Altaf, M. S. Halim, N. Rajagopalan, and A. Javed Khan. 2014. "Aspiration in Injections: Should We Continue or Abandon the Practice?" *F1000Research* 3: 157. https://doi.org/10.12688/f1000research.1113.3.

Shaffer, J. 2016. "Neuroplasticity and Clinical Practice: Building Brain Power for Health." *Frontiers in Psychology* 7: 1118. https://doi.org/10.3389/fpsyg.2016.01118.

Shang, S. Z., W. Zhao, J. G. Tang, X. M. Xu, H. D. Sun, J. X. Pu, Z. H. Liu, M. M. Miao, Y. K. Chen, and G. Y. Yang. 2016. "Antiviral Sesquiterpenes from Leaves of Nicotiana tabacum." *Fitoterapia* 108: 1–4. https://doi.org/10.1016/j.fitote.2015.11.004.

Shannon, S., N. Lewis, H. Lee, and S. Hughes. 2019. "Cannabidiol in Anxiety and Sleep: A Large Case Series." *Permanente Journal* 23: 18–41. https://doi.org/10.7812/TPP/18-041.

Shi, H., Y. Zuo, S. Navaz, A. Harbaugh, C. K. Hoy, A. A. Gandhi, G. Sule, S. Yalavarthi, K. Gockman, J. A. Madison, J. Wang, M. Zuo, Y. Shi, M. D. Maile, J. S. Knight, and Y. Kanthi. 2022. "Endothelial Cell–Activating Antibodies in COVID-19." *Arthritis & Rheumatology* 74: 1132–38. https://doi.org/10.1002/art.42094

Shi, Z., and C. A. Puyo. 2020. "N-acetylcysteine to Combat COVID-19: An Evidence Review." *Therapeutics and Clinical Risk Management* 16: 1047–55. https://doi.org/10.2147/TCRM.S273700.

Shin, T. Y., S. H. Kim, S. H. Kim, Y. K. Kim, H. J. Park, B. S. Chae, H. J. Jung, and H. M. Kim. 2000. "Inhibitory Effect of Mast Cell-Mediated Immediate-Type Allergic Reactions in Rats by Perilla frutescens." *Immunopharmacology and Immunotoxicology* 22, no. 3: 489–500. https://doi.org/10.3109/08923970009026007.

Siddiqui, M. Z. 2011. "Boswellia serrata, a Potential Antiinflammatory Agent: An Overview." *Indian Journal of Pharmaceutical Sciences* 73, no. 3: 255–61. https://doi.org/10.4103/0250-474X.93507.

Silvagno, F., A. Vernone, and G. P. Pescarmona. 2020. "The Role of Glutathione in Protecting against the Severe Inflammatory Response Triggered by COVID-19." *Antioxidants* (Basel) 9, no. 7: 624. https://doi.org/10.3390/antiox9070624.

Silveira, D., J. M. Prieto-Garcia, F. Boylan, O. Estrada, Y. M. Fonseca-Bazzo, C. M. Jamal, P. O. Magalhães, E. O. Pereira, M. Tomczyk, and M. Heinrich. 2020. "COVID-19: Is There Evidence for the Use of Herbal Medicines as Adjuvant Symptomatic Therapy?" *Frontiers in Pharmacology* 11: 581840. https://doi.org/10.3389/fphar.2020.581840.

Simmons-Boyce, Joanne L., and Winston F. Tinto. 2007. "Steroidal Saponins and Sapogenins from the Agavaceae Family." *Natural Product Communications* 2, no. 1: 99–114.

Sims, Matthew, William Beaumont Hospitals. 2022. "Study of Immunomodulation Using Naltrexone and Ketamine for COVID-19 (SINK COVID-19)." Clinical trial report published on the US National Library of Medicine website, January 26, 2022. Identifier no. NCT04365985.

Singh, R. K., H. W. Chang, D. Yan, K. M. Lee, D. Ucmak, K. Wong, M. Abrouk, et al. 2017. "Influence of Diet on the Gut Microbiome and Implications for Human Health." *Journal of Translational Medicine* 15, no. 1: 73. https://doi.org/10.1186/s12967-017-1175-y.

Song, Eric, Christopher M. Bartley, Ryan D. Chow, Thomas T. Ngo, Ruoyi Jiang, Colin R. Zamecnik, Ravi Dandekar, et al. 2021. "Divergent and Self-Reactive Immune Responses in the CNS of COVID-19 Patients with Neurological Symptoms." *Cell Reports: Medicine* 2, no. 5: 100288.

Sonnenburg, J., and E. Sonnenburg. 2015. "Gut Feelings: 'The Second Brain' in Our Gastrointestinal Systems." *Scientific American,* May 1, 2015. From *The Good Gut: Taking Control of Your Mood and Your Long-Term Health*.

Sorrentino, Matthew. 2012. "An Update on Statin Alternatives and Adjunct." *Journal of Clinical Lipidology* 7, no. 6: 721–30.

Sozańska, B. 2019. "Raw Cow's Milk and Its Protective Effect on Allergies and Asthma." *Nutrients* 11, no. 2: 469. https://doi.org/10.3390/nu11020469.

Stamets, P. A. 1999. *Mycomedicinals: An Informational Treatise on Mushrooms.* Whistler, Canada: Mycomedia.

Stamets, P. and H. Zwickey. 2014. "Medicinal Mushrooms: Ancient Remedies Meet Modern Science." *Integrative Medicine* 13, no. 1 (February): 46–47.

Stelwagen, K., E. Carpenter, B. Haigh, A. Hodgkinson, and T. T. Wheeler. 2009. "Immune Components of Bovine Colostrum and Milk." *Journal of Animal Science* 87, no. 13 (suppl): 3–9. https://doi.org/10.2527/jas.2008-1377.

Subroto, Edy, and Rossi Indiarto. 2020. "Bioactive Monolaurin as an Antimicrobial and Its Potential to Improve the Immune System and against COVID-19: A Review." *Food Research* 4: 2355–65. https://doi.org/10.26656/fr.2017.4(6).324.

Sukhatme, V. P., A. M. Reiersen, S. J. Vayttaden, and V. V. Sukhatme. 2021. Fluvoxamine: A Review of Its Mechanism of Action and Its Role in COVID-19." *Frontiers in Pharmacology* 12: 652688. https://doi.org/10.3389/fphar.2021.652688.

Survivor Corps Facebook Group. 2021. Vaccine Poll. Facebook, February 27, 2021.

Swank, Zoe, Yasmeen Senussi, Zachary Manickas-Hill, Xu G. Yu, Jonathan Z. Li, Galit Alter, and David R. Walt. 2022. "Persistent Circulating Severe Acute Respiratory Syndrome Coronavirus-2 Spike Is Associated with Post-Acute Coronavirus Disease 2019 Sequelae." *Clinical Infectious Diseases* ciac722. https://doi.org/10.1093/cid/ciac722.

Szabo, A. 2015. "Psychedelics and Immunomodulation: Novel Approaches and Therapeutic Opportunities." *Frontiers in Immunology* 6: 358. https://doi.org/10.3389/fimmu.2015.00358.

Taquet, Maxime Geddes, John R. Husain, Masud Luciano, Sierra Harrison, and Paul J. Harrison. 2021. "6-month Neurological and Psychiatric Outcomes in 236 379 Survivors of COVID-19: A Retrospective Cohort Study Using Electronic Health Records." *Lancet Psychiatry* 8, no. 5: 416–27. https://doi.org/10.1016/S2215-0366(21)00084-5.

Tariq, Asma, Rana Muhammad Mateen, Muhammad Sohail Afzal, and Mahjabeen Saleem. 2020. "Paromomycin: A Potential Dual Targeted Drug Effectively Inhibits Both Spike (S1) and Main Protease of COVID-19." *International Journal of Infectious Diseases* 98: 166–75.

Tashkin, D. P., and R. P. Murray. 2009. "Smoking Cessation in Chronic Obstructive Pulmonary Disease." *Respiratory Medicine* 103, no. 7: 963–74.

Theoharides, T. C., C. Cholevas, K. Polyzoidis, and A. Politis. 2021. "Long-COVID Syndrome-Associated Brain Fog and Chemofog: Luteolin to the Rescue." *Biofactors* 47, no. 2: 232–41. https://doi.org/10.1002/biof.1726.

Thimmulappa, R. K., K. K. Mudnakudu-Nagaraju, and C. Shivamallu, et al. 2021. "Antiviral and Immunomodulatory Activity of Curcumin: A Case for Prophylactic Therapy for COVID-19." *Heliyon* 7, no. 2: e06350. https://doi.org/10.1016/j.heliyon.2021.e06350.

Thomas, Robert, Jeffrey Aldous, Rachel Forsyth, Angel M. Chater, and Madeleine Williams. 2021. "The Influence of a Blend of Probiotic Lactobacillus and Prebiotic Inulin on the Duration and Severity of Symptoms among Individuals with Covid-19." *Infectious Diseases: Research and Treatment* 5, no. 1: 1–12. https://doi.org/10.29011/2577-1515.100182.

Thompson, C., and A. Szabo. 2020. "Psychedelics as a Novel Approach to Treating Autoimmune Conditions." *Immunology Letters* 228: 45–54. https://doi.org/10.1016/j.imlet.2020.10.001.

Thomson, H. 2021. "Children with Long Covid." *New Scientist* 249, no. 3323: 10–11. https://doi.org/10.1016/S0262-4079(21)00303-1.

Tiwari, M. 2017. "The Role of Serratiopeptidase in the Resolution of Inflammation." *Asian Journal of Pharmaceutical Science* 12, no. 3: 209–15. https://doi.org/10.1016/j.ajps.2017.01.003.

Townsend, L., A. H. Dyer, P. McCluskey, K. O'Brien, J. Dowds, E. Laird, C. Bannan, et al. 2021. "Investigating the Relationship between Vitamin D and Persistent Symptoms

Following SARS-CoV-2 Infection." *Nutrients* 13, no. 7: 2430. https://doi.org/10.3390/nu13072430.

Trimble, M., and D. Hesdorffer. 2017. "Music and the Brain: The Neuroscience of Music and Musical Appreciation." *BJPsych International* 14, no. 2: 28–31. https://doi.org/10.1192/s2056474000001720.

Tu, Y., Y. Zhang, Y. Li, et al. 2021. "Post-Traumatic Stress Symptoms in COVID-19 Survivors: A Self-Report and Brain Imaging Follow-Up Study." *Molecular Psychiatry* 26: 7475–80. https://doi.org/10.1038/s41380-021-01223-w.

Turner, J. S., A. Day, W. B. Alsoussi, Z. Liu, J A O'Halloran, R. M. Presti, B. K. Patterson, S. P. J. Whelan, A. H. Ellebedy, and P. A. Mudd. 2021. "SARS-CoV-2 Viral RNA Shedding for More Than 87 Days in an Individual with an Impaired CD8+ T Cell Response." *Frontiers in Immunology* 11: 618402. https://doi.org/10.3389/fimmu.2020.618402.

Ubillas, R., S. D. Jolad, R. C. Bruening, M. R. Kernan, S. R. King, D. F. Sesin, M. Barrett, et al. 1994. "SP-303, an Antiviral Oligomeric Proanthocyanidin from the Latex of Croton lechleri (Sangre de Drago)." *Phytomedicine* 1, no. 2: 77–106. https://doi.org/10.1016/S0944-7113(11)80026-7.

UK Essays. 2013. "Effect of Cigarette Smoke on Mold Growth." UK Essays, November 2013.

Umesh, A., K. Pranay, R. C. Pandey, et al. 2022. "Evidence Mapping and Review of Long-COVID and Its Underlying Pathophysiological Mechanism." *Infection* 50, no. 5. https://doi.org/10.1007/s15010-022-01835-6.

University of Birmingham. 2020. "Scientists 'Re-train' Immune System to Prevent Attack of Healthy Cells." ScienceDaily (online), June 9, 2020.

University of Illinois at Chicago. 2019. "Technique boosts omega 3 fatty acid levels in brain 100 fold." ScienceDaily (online), January 8, 2019.

Vairo, G. L., S. J. Miller, N. M. McBrier, and W. E. Buckley. 2009. "Systematic Review of Efficacy for Manual Lymphatic Drainage Techniques in Sports Medicine and Rehabilitation: An Evidence-Based Practice Approach." *Journal of Manual and Manipulative Therapy* 17, no. 3: e80–89. https://doi.org/10.1179/jmt.2009.17.3.80E.

van der Kroon, C. 1996. *The Golden Fountain: The Complete Guide to Urine Therapy.* Chicago: Wishland.

Vaziri-Harami, R., and P. Delkash. 2021. "Can L-carnitine Reduce Post-COVID-19 Fatigue?" *Annals of Medicine and Surgery* (London) 73.103145. https://doi.org/10.1016/j.amsu.2021.103145.

Veloso, T. R., F. Oechslin, Y. A. Que, P. Moreillon, J. M. Entenza, and S. Mancini. 2015. "Aspirin Plus Ticlopidine Prevented Experimental Endocarditis due to Enterococcus faecalis and Streptococcus gallolyticus." *Pathogens and Disease* 73, no. 8: ftv060. https://doi.org/10.1093/femspd/ftv060.

Veness, Bianca. N.d. "How I Use Pacing to Manage ME/CFS." ME/CFS and Fibromyalgia Self-Help website.

Venkatesan, Priya. 2022. "Do Vaccines Protect from Long Covid?" *Lancet Respiratory Medicine* 10, no. 3: e30.

Verity, Robert, et al. 2020. "Estimates of the Severity of Coronavirus Disease 2019: A Model-Based Analysis." *The Lancet Infectious Diseases* 20, no. 6: 669–77.

Vetvicka, V., and J. Vetvickova. 2011. Immune Enhancing Effects of WB365, a Novel Combination of Ashwagandha (Withania somnifera) and Maitake (Grifola frondosa) Extracts." *North American Journal of Medicine and Science* 3, no. 7: 320–24. https://doi.org/10.4297/najms.2011.3320.

V'kovski, P., A. Kratzel, S. Steiner, et al. 2021. "Coronavirus Biology and Replication: Implications for SARS-CoV-2." *Nature Reviews Microbiology* 19: 155–70. https://doi.org/10.1038/s41579-020-00468-6.

Waheed W., M. E. Carey, S. R. Tandan, and R. Tandan. 2021. "Post COVID-19 Vaccine Small Fiber Neuropathy." *Muscle & Nerve* 64, no. 1:E1–E2. https://doi.org/10.1002/mus.27251.

Wang, F. Y., S. Y. He, Z. J. Zhang, L. F. He, X. W. Chen, and T. Teng. 2011. "Analyses of Anti-HIV Type 1 Activity of a Small CCR5 Peptide Antagonist." *AIDS Research and Human Retroviruses* 27, no. 10: 1111–15. https://doi.org/10.1089/AID.2010.0303.

Wang, H., Z. Yuan, M. A. Pavel, et al. 2021. "The Role of High Cholesterol in Age-Related COVID19 Lethality." bioRxiv preprint. https://doi.org/10.1101/2020.05.09.086249.

Wang, K. Y., L. Tull, E. Cooper, N. Wang, and D. Liu. 2013. "Recombinant Protein Production of Earthworm Lumbrokinase for Potential Antithrombotic Application." *Evidence-Based Complementary and Alternative Medicine* 2013: 783971. https://doi.org/10.1155/2013/783971.

Wang, L., Y. Zhao, Y. Yang, et al. 2017. "Allergens in Red Ginseng Extract Induce the Release of Mediators Associated with Anaphylactoid Reactions." *Journal of Translational Medicine* 15: 148. https://doi.org/10.1186/s12967-017-1249-x.

Wang, N., S. Han, R. Liu, L. Meng, H. He, Y. Zhang, C. Wang, Y. Lv, J. Wang, X. Li, et al. 2020. "Chloroquine and Hydroxychloroquine as ACE2 Blockers to Inhibit Viropexis of 2019-nCoV Spike Pseudotyped Virus." *Phytomedicine* 79: 153333. https://doi.org/10.1016/j.phymed.2020.153333.

Wang, S., P. Ma, S. Zhang, et al. 2020. "Fasting Blood Glucose at Admission Is an Independent Predictor for 28-Day Mortality in Patients with Covid-19 without Previous Diagnosis of Diabetes: A Multi-Centre Retrospective Study." *Diabetologia* 63: 2102–11. https://doi.org/10.1007/s00125-020-05209-1.

Waxenbaum, J. A., V. Reddy, and M. Varacallo. 2021. "Anatomy, Autonomic Nervous System." StatPearls (online). Treasure Island, Fla.: StatPearls Publishing. Updated July 29, 2021.

Weinbroum, A. A. 2021. "Perspectives of Ketamine Use in COVID-19 Patients." *Journal of Korean Medical Science* 36, no. 4: e28. https://doi.org/10.3346/jkms.2021.36.e28.

Weinstock, L. B., J. B. Brook, A. S. Walters, A. Goris, L. B. Afrin, and G. J. Molderings. 2021. "Mast Cell Activation Symptoms Are Prevalent in Long-COVID." *International Journal of Infectious Diseases* 112: 217–26. https://doi.org/10.1016/j.ijid.2021.09.043.

Weisblum, Y., F. Schmidt, F. Zhang, J. DaSilva, D. Poston, J. C. Lorenzi, F. Muecksch, et al. 2020. "Escape from Neutralizing Antibodies by SARS-CoV-2 Spike Protein Variants." *eLife* 9: e61312. https://doi.org/10.7554/eLife.61312.

Wieland, L.S., V. Piechotta, T. Feinberg, et al. 2021. "Elderberry for Prevention and Treatment of Viral Respiratory Illnesses: A Systematic Review." *BMC Complementary Medicine and Therapies* 21: 112. https://doi.org/10.1186/s12906-021-03283-5.

Wijaya, I., R. Andhika, I. Huang, A. Purwiga, and K. Y. Budiman. 2021. "The Effects of Aspirin on the Outcome of COVID-19: A Systematic Review and Meta-Analysis." *Clinical Epidemiology and Global Health* 12: 100883. https://doi.org/10.1016/j.cegh.2021.100883.

Winkler, John, and Sanjoy Ghosh. 2018. "Therapeutic Potential of Fulvic Acid in Chronic Inflammatory Diseases and Diabetes." *Journal of Diabetes Research* 2018, no. 5391014. https://doi.org/10.1155/2018/5391014.

Witt, C. M., R. Lüdtke, S. N. Willich. 2010. "Homeopathic Treatment of Patients with Migraine: A Prospective Observational Study with a 2-Year Follow-Up Period." *Journal of Alternative and Complementary Medicine* 16, no. 4: 347–55. https://doi.org/10.1089/acm.2009.0376.

Wolpe, J. 1987. "Carbon Dioxide Inhalation Treatments of Neurotic Anxiety. An Overview." *Journal of Nervous and Mental Disease* 175, no. 3: 129–33. https://doi.org/10.1097/00005053-198703000-00001.

World Wildlife Fund. N.d. "How Many Species Are We Losing?" World Wildlife Fund website.

——. 2020. *Living Planet Report 2020: Bending the Curve of Biodiversity Loss.* Eds. R. E. A. Almond, M. Grooten, and T. Petersen. Gland, Switzerland: World Wildlife Fund.

Wostyn, P. 2021. "COVID-19 and Chronic Fatigue Syndrome: Is the Worst Yet to Come?" *Medical Hypotheses* 146: 110469. doi10.1016/j.mehy.2020.110469.

Wu Zhang, X, and Y. Leng Yap. 2004. "Structural Similarity between HIV-1 gp41 and SARS-CoV S2 Proteins Suggests an Analogous Membrane Fusion Mechanism." *Journal of Molecular Structure: THEOCHEM* 677, no. 1: 73–76. https://doi.org/10.1016/j.theochem.2004.02.018.

Wu, H., and E. Wu. 2012. "The Role of Gut Microbiota in Immune Homeostasis and Autoimmunity." *Gut Microbes* 1: 4–14.

Wusteman, M., D. G. Wight, and M. Elia. 1990. "Protein Metabolism after Injury with Turpentine: A Rat Model for Clinical Trauma." *American Journal of Physiology* 259, no. 6, pt. 1: E763–69. https://doi.org/10.1152/ajpendo.1990.259.6.E763.

Xiao, Zijian, Qing Ye, Xiaomei Duan, and Tao Xiang. 2021. "Network Pharmacology Reveals That Resveratrol Can Alleviate COVID-19-Related Hyperinflammation." *Disease Markers* 2021, no. 4129993. https://doi.org/10.1155/2021/4129993.

Xiao-yl, C., L. Yuan, L. Wei, M. Wang, and L. Yi-xiong. 2014. "Content Analysis of Shikimic Acid in the Masson Pine Needles and Antiplatelet-Aggregating Activity." *International Journal of Agricultural Science and Technology* 2, no. 4: 110. https://doi.org/10.14355/ijast.2014.0204.03.

Yang, C. R., Y. Zhang, M. R. Jacob, S. I. Khan, Y. J. Zhang, and X. C. Li. 2006. "Antifungal Activity of C-27 Steroidal Saponins." *Antimicrobial Agents and Chemotherapy* 50, no. 5: 1710–14.

Yang, Ming-Wei, Feng Chen, Ding-Jun Zhu, Jia-Zhu Li, Jin-Ling Zhu, Wei Zeng, Shi-Lin Qu, and Yun Zhang. 2020. "Clinical Efficacy of Matrine and Sodium Chloride Injection in Treatment of 40 Cases of COVID-19. *Zhongguo Zhong Yao Za Zh* 45, no. 10.

Yang, Y., Y. Wu, X. Meng, et al. 2022. "SARS-CoV-2 Membrane Protein Causes the Mitochondrial Apoptosis and Pulmonary Edema via Targeting BOK." *Cell Death & Differentiation* 29: 1395–1408. https://doi.org/10.1038/s41418-022-00928-x.

Yeoh, Y. K., T. Zuo, G. C. Lui, et al. 2021. "Gut Microbiota Composition Reflects Disease Severity and Dysfunctional Immune Responses In Patients with COVID-19." *Gut* 70: 698–706.

Yepes-Pérez, A. F., O. Herrera-Calderon, and J. Quintero-Saumeth. 2022. "Uncaria tomentosa (Cat's Claw): A Promising Herbal Medicine against SARS-CoV-2/ACE-2 Junction and SARS-CoV-2 Spike Protein Based on Molecular Modeling." *Journal of Biomolecular Structures and Dynamics* 40, no. 5: 2227–43. https://doi.org/10.1080/07391102.2020.1837676.

Yokosuka, A., Y. Mimaki, M. Kuroda, and Y. Sashida. 2000. A New Steroidal Saponin from the Leaves of Agave americana." *Planta Medica* 66, no. 4: 393–96. https://doi.org/10.1055/s-2000-8546.

Yousefi, H., L. Mashouri, S. C. Okpechi, N. Alahari, and S. K. Alahari. 2021. "Repurposing Existing Drugs for the Treatment of COVID-19/SARS-CoV-2 Infection: A Review Describing Drug Mechanisms of Action." *Biochemical Pharmacology* 183: 114296. https://doi.org/10.1016/j.bcp.2020.114296.

Yu, S., Y. Zhu, J. Xu, et al. 2021. "Glycyrrhizic Acid Exerts Inhibitory Activity against the Spike Protein of SARS-CoV-2." *Phytomedicine* 85: 153364. https://doi.org/10.1016/j.phymed.2020.153364.

Zalta, E., ed. 2006. "The Uncertainty Principle." In *Stanford Encyclopedia of Philosophy.* Stanford, Calif: Metaphysics Research Lab, Stanford University.

Zamani, B., S. M. Moeini Taba, and M. Shayestehpour. 2021. "Systemic Lupus Erythematosus Manifestation Following COVID-19: A Case Report." *Journal of Medical Case Reports* 15: 29. https://doi.org/10.1186/s13256-020-02582-8.

Zeberg, H., and S. Pääbo. 2020. "The Major Genetic Risk Factor for Severe COVID-19 Is Inherited from Neanderthals." *Nature* 587: 610–612. https://doi.org/10.1038/s41586-020-2818-3.

Zhan, Y., W. Ta, W. Tang, et al. 2021. "Potential Antiviral Activity of Isorhamnetin against SARS-CoV-2 Spike Pseudotyped Virus In Vitro." *Drug Development Research* 82, no. 8: 1124–30. https://doi.org/10.1002/ddr.21815.

Zhang, J., T. Xiao, Y. Cai, C. L. Lavine, H. Peng, H. Zhu, K. Anand, et al. 2021. "Membrane Fusion and Immune Evasion by the Spike Protein of SARS-CoV-2 Delta Variant." bioRxiv preprint. https://doi.org/10.1101/2021.08.17.456689.

Zhang, X., K. M. Haney, A. C. Richardson, et al. 2010. "Anibamine, a Natural Product CCR5 Antagonist, as a Novel Lead for the Development of Anti-prostate Cancer Agents." *Bioorganic and Medicinal Chemistry Letters* 20, no. 15: 4627–30. https://doi.org/10.1016/j.bmcl.2010.06.003.

Zhou, Y., K. Gilmore, S. Ramirez, et al. 2021. "In Vitro Efficacy of Artemisinin-Based Treatments against SARS-CoV-2." *Scientific Reports* 11, no. 1: 14571. https://doi.org/10.1038/s41598-021-93361-y.

Zhou, Y., Y. Hou, J. Shen, R. Mehra, A. Kallianpur, D. A. Culver, et al. 2020. "A Network Medicine Approach to Investigation and Population-Based Validation of Disease Manifestations and Drug Repurposing for COVID-19." *PLOS Biology* 18, no. 11: e3000970. https://doi.org/10.1371/journal.pbio.3000970.

Zielińska, A., and I. Nowak. 2017. "Abundance of Active Ingredients in Sea-Buckthorn Oil." *Lipids in Health and Disease* 16, no. 1: 95. https://doi.org/10.1186/s12944-017-0469-7.

Zou, W., Z. Xiao, X. Wen, J. Luo, S. Chen, Z. Cheng, D. Xiang, J. Hu, and J. He. 2016. "The Anti-inflammatory Effect of Andrographis paniculata (Burm. f.) Nees on Pelvic Inflammatory Disease in Rats through Down-Regulation of the NF-κB Pathway." *BMC Complementary and Alternative Medicine* 16, no. 1: 483. https://doi.org/10.1186/s12906-016-1466-5.

Index